BEYOND BIRTHING IMPOSSIBILITIES

My VBAC Journey

Shola Bankole, MD

ISBN: 979-8-9898468-0-1

DISCLAIMER

This book is for sharing my VBAC journey and not intended to provide medical advice. You should always consult with your physician/medical specialists. While the author and editors have taken reasonable steps to ensure accuracy of Information, we encourage you to consult with your physician during every step of your pregnancy process. The author specifically disclaims any liability for omissions or errors found in this book.

Published by:

BankyEstates LLC

Beyondbirthingimpossibilities@gmail.com

CONTENTS

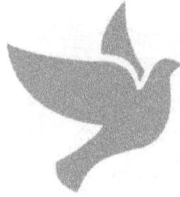

DEDICATION

I dedicate this book to my late father, Pa Olugbemiga James. Thank you for giving me the greatest gift of all, by introducing me to Jesus Christ. A favorite phrase you commonly shared was that the best inheritance you can give any one of us is an education. Thank you for your investment in me. I love and honor you Dad. Continue to rest in the sweet bosom of Father Abraham.

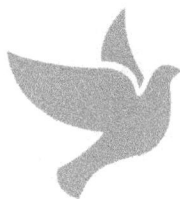

ACKNOWLEDGEMENTS

The inspiration to write this book was given by God the Father, Son, and Holy Spirit. Thus, I give all the glory to God, for without God, there would be no book.

Harriet Atsegbua, whom I trusted with this project. Thank you for helping make this vision a reality. Thank you for your incredible gift of writing and skills that were poured into this book.

My mother and father, Mr. and Mrs. Santana, thank you for all your prayers, love, and support.

My parents in the Lord, Pastors Yomi and Bisi Oshikoya and Pastors Akin and Kenny Olubiyi. Thank you for all your prayers, love, leadership, and mentorship.

To my siblings, I love you all. Thank you for your continuous love and support.

To my husband, Pastor Olasunkanmi Isaac Bankole, words are not enough to express my love and appreciation. This book would not have been possible without you. Thank you for bringing out the best in me and helping in the fulfilment of God's purpose in our lives. You are a phenomenal husband, father, and engineer, and I love and appreciate you dearly.

To my children, Enoch, Elijah, Emmanuel, and Ezekiel. You are the best gifts and I love you all.

Thank you and God bless you.

Thank you to my readers for taking the time to read this book,

God bless you.

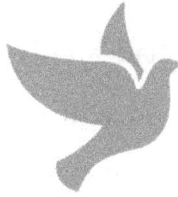

PREFACE

"Every good gift and every perfect gift is from above, and cometh down from the Father of lights, with whom is no variableness, neither shadow of turning." — James 1:7 (KJV)

I wrote this book primarily to share my experience of having two vaginal births after two cesarean sections and not necessarily to advocate for one method over another. As a young woman who nurtured the hopes of becoming a mother, I always expected that I would give birth vaginally.

After having my first baby via a cesarean section, I had a long road to recovery and given how demanding my job is and how quickly I had to return to work, I felt as though I would have bounced back a lot quicker if I had not had to endure a surgical procedure. Thus, at that juncture, my desire for a vaginal birth was born.

With my second baby, I had another cesarean section and a similar uphill climb as I did with my first delivery. I knew I wanted more children and did not want to go through painful birthing experiences and equally challenging healing processes in a bid to complete my family.

Thus, I started my research into the possibility of having a successful vaginal birth after a cesarean section. Once I knew it could be achieved and was cleared for the process by a team of trusted medical experts, I began the journey by faith. Every mother's journey is unique and no form of birthing a child is superior to another. The best method for any mother is the method her medical team believes is safe and one that has a healthy mother and baby as the goal.

Thus, my intent is not to advocate for a method that might be unsafe or one that could jeopardize the health or life of the mother or baby.

I had a desire that had gone unfulfilled and knowing that there was a possibility I could fulfill it with the help of God and an amazing medical team behind me, I decided to give it a try. I was able to successfully have two vaginal births after two cesarean sections.

My goal is to let women just like myself who have the same desire know that the option of having a vaginal birth after a cesarean section is a possibility. Importantly, I hope that beyond evaluating your options, that when you pick up this book, you realize how amazing your body is to uniquely carry a baby from conception to birth, and that you understand that you are not defined by your birthing method, but that your identity lies in being known and loved by God.

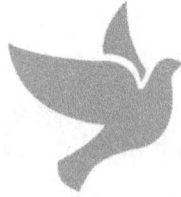

INTRODUCTION

Prior to having my first child, I never considered comparing birth notes or swapping birth stories with other mothers. I assumed I would get all the information I needed from my obstetrician, and I also somehow assumed that I would instinctively know exactly how to proceed.

Additionally, I was having what you would say was an easy pregnancy, so I expected my birthing process to be just as hitch free. As it turned out, I did not get all the information I needed from my doctor because I truly did not even know what questions to ask in the first place, and my doctor in turn only asked textbook questions that didn't quite elicit answers that went beyond the norm.

The truth is sufficient education is not always provided when it comes to birthing babies. Many women have assumptions about the process, but those assumptions often end up being far from reality. That was certainly the case in my experience.

I planned to show up with my makeup flawlessly done, so I would be ready for my photo op when the baby popped out after a few pushes. I was underprepared for what would follow and in retrospect, my experience was a result of my obstetrician only asking the routine questions and responding to the basic questions I posed in return because I did not quite know what to ask. In general, I found the entire process quite daunting even though I am a practicing emergency room resident physician.

I did not take any prenatal classes due to my busy resident schedule. My thought was also that since I am a physician and have delivered multiple babies, there would be really nothing new to learn in these classes for me. But now I know, and I encourage you to take all prenatal classes offered online or in your area because you will learn new things. It is quite the contradiction.

I expected an easy birthing process with beautifully captured photographs, yet I was overwhelmed by the information and burdened by questions I did not quite know how to frame. Thus, what I expected would be an easy process ended up in a cesarean section followed by a long recovery. With my second pregnancy, I felt a bit better prepared but also had a cesarean section then. In many cases, cesarean sections are lifesaving and absolutely necessary, but after having two cesarean sections that were followed by long recoveries, I began to challenge the procedure and ponder whether I could have birthed my babies differently.

Knowing I wanted more children and not wanting to endure any more surgeries, my questions led me to begin seeking out women who had vaginal births after cesarean sections (VBACs) with a desire to hear their stories and ask questions. I reasoned that if God designed humans perfectly and created the birth canal, then He definitely had intentions for its use. Thus, as I began to swap stories with other mothers, I noticed that the rates of cesarean sections (now at 32.1% between 1997-2021, according to Statista.com)[1] far outpaced vaginal births.

---

[1] "Percentage of all live births by Cesarean delivery in the United States from 1997 to 2021," Statista.com, **https://www.statista.com/statistics/184079/us-hospital-stays-with-cesarean-section-procedures-since-1997/**

I realized that with American society being so litigious and given the long years of training obstetricians have to endure, opting to perform cesarean sections has become quite popular to help doctors avoid legal challenges. Further, cesarean sections are more financially rewarding for medical practices.

As I journeyed on, my quest led me to seek out narratives that reflected my desire. I pinned my hope to the anchor scripture, *"For with God nothing shall be impossible"* (Luke 1:37 KJV). Thus, I began a faith walk and went on to have two more pregnancies that culminated in vaginal births. As a physician I value the blessing of scientific advances, cesarean sections being one of them. This book does not decry them, as they are absolutely required in many instances to save the lives of the mother and baby. But I wanted a different experience and drew on my faith to have vaginal births after two cesarean sections. Thus, the most important message my book seeks to deliver is that it is possible to experience a vaginal delivery even after cesarean sections and I want women who desire this to ask questions and explore the possibility.[2]

---

[2] Emily Oster and W. Spencer McClelland, "Why the C-Section Rate Is So High," *The Atlantic*, October 17, 2019,
https://www.theatlantic.com/ideas/archive/2019/10/c-section-rate-high/600172/

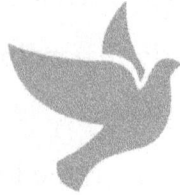

CHAPTER 1

MY FAITH AND CONFESSION

Now faith is the substance of things hoped for, the evidence of things not seen. — Hebrews 11:1 (NKJV)

Going through the process of wanting a vaginal birth after two cesarean sections made me engage in some important soul-searching exercises. I had to ask some critical questions about whom and what I truly believed in. Since I still wanted another baby and hoped for a vaginal birth, I knew that it would require me to truly stretch my faith and put what I truly believed to the test.

I had to examine my faith in God and question if the miracles I knew God was capable of performing applied to my desire for a natural birth.

Yes, I knew God was able to do the impossible, but did that apply to my situation? It wasn't as though I didn't have options or as though I were trapped. I had an option or so it seemed, which would be another cesarean section, but I stubbornly wanted to experience having my husband "catch" our next baby and be back on my feet in no time at all. Hey, don't get me wrong, recovery after a vaginal birth isn't always necessarily easy, but it at least typically doesn't have the potential complications from surgery (C-section).

Believing for a vaginal birth seemed like an uphill battle but I had a good deal of support as I made my ascent. I had the testimonies of others who had walked that path with success and that gave me hope that God was able. Also, I spent a good deal of time listening to the testimonies of others and trying to glean from their blessings and testimonies. I reasoned that if God could give these women the experience of having vaginal births after cesarean sections, then He was more than able to do the same for me.

Prime amongst the testimonies I listened to was that of the General Overseer of my church, the Redeemed Christian Church of God (RCCG), Pastor E.A. Adeboye and his wife, Mrs. Adeboye, whom we fondly refer to as Daddy G.O. and Mommy G.O., with "G.O." standing for General Overseer.

I connected to the testimonies of my Daddy and Mommy G.O. They shared how Mommy G.O. was able to have a vaginal delivery by the grace of God after three cesarean sections 44 years ago, by completely leaning on God's faithfulness.

In addition to listening to their testimony, I had to hold on to the truth of the word of God. I speak here of truth because I had to counter the lies that kept gnawing at me and telling me my desires were not feasible. My anchor scripture became Luke 1:37 (KJV), *"with God nothing shall be impossible."* I kept meditating on this scripture and believing that the breadth of what God was capable of doing included the promise of a vaginal birth in spite of the statistics that were not in my favor.

All signs pointed in the direction of another caesarean section when I was expecting my third baby.

I went over the drill in my head: show up, change into my hospital gown, and be wheeled off into the operating room to be cut open. I remembered being too sore to hold my babies after my previous births and peeking at them as they were held up for my viewing pleasure. I knew for a fact that I didn't want to repeat that sequence.

So, tempting as it was to rehearse what seemed familiar and what was the only reference I had as far as childbirth was concerned, I kept challenging myself to keep my mind renewed and to think differently. Thus, my journey of faith was twofold, unlearning old narratives and embracing the new, which was meditating on the truth of God's word regarding my desire for a vaginal birth.

I also had to learn to be positive. I made it a point to heavily research statistics about vaginal births after cesarean sections (VBACs) with some reservation, refusing to allow the facts to replace the truth I was clinging to. I did my research extensively and made sure I was educated. The facts did not negate the truth that I believed in.

Based on the Natality Data Files in the National Vital Statistics System (derived from birth certificates for all births occurring in the United States), the rate of VBACs was 12.4% in 2016. By 2017, that number saw a slight uptick to 12.8% and then reached 13.3% in 2018. The increase in these numbers from 2016 until 2018 was seen mostly in women in their twenties and thirties and in women of all races and Hispanic-origin groups except non-Hispanic Native Hawaiian or other Pacific Islander women.[3]

Once I made up my mind that I wanted my next baby to arrive vaginally as opposed to through a caesarean section, my next task involved finding a reputable and experienced physician who would guide me through the process. I started searching for a doctor after conception, but the search process for finding a VBAC-friendly physician can begin as early as the preconception stage. It was a very difficult and challenging time as I did not want to settle for just any physician.

---

[3] Michelle J.K. Osterman, "Recent Trends in Vaginal Birth After Cesarean Delivery: United States, 2016–2018," NCHS Data Brief No. 359, March 2020, **https://www.cdc.gov/nchs/products/databriefs/db359.htm**

During my search, my choices were slim because most of the physicians and offices I called were not accepting new patients or were not taking patients who had already had two cesarean sections. But I give thanks to God for the physician He brought my way through this process.

In most instance, many physicians are uncomfortable with women attempting vaginal births after having a previous caesarean section. There are a number of risks factors involved with the process, such as a uterine rupture, which though life threatening is rare and occurs in less than 1% of women who attempt a VBAC.[4]

The danger with a trial of labor after cesarean (TOLAC) is that it could result in uterine ruptures due to a previous cesarean scar on the uterus reopening, which might cause severe bleeding, loss of the fetus, and also lead to a surgical removal of the uterus, which is a complete hysterectomy and can be fatal if not urgently realized.

[4] Mayo Clinic, "Labor and Delivery, Postpartum Care," December 03, 2022, https://www.mayoclinic.org/healthy-lifestyle/labor-and-delivery/in-depth/vbac/art-20044869

The health complications are why doctors shy away from the practice and I understood this going in. However, I knew that a successful vaginal delivery would involve far fewer complications than a cesarean section and that absent any complications I would be back on my feet in no time at all (compared to the process of recovering from surgery).

Thus, I began my search for a doctor. In my current locale, I was unable to find a doctor as most physicians who perform VBACs were fully booked and not accepting any more patients. I was quite bummed when I discovered that my options for a physician were pretty slim as I was already six weeks along and to be honest, it was quite distressing. So, as my pregnancy progressed, I knew I would have to cast a wider net.

I began to search outside of the city I resided in and began to look at surrounding cities that had a teaching hospital or access to adequate resources should I end up with a failed trial of labor and require an emergency cesarean section. Initially, there was some concern with the process, as I was told I had an anthropoid pelvis that would make it challenging to have a vaginal delivery.

There are four types of pelvic shapes: gynecoid (most favorable for vaginal births), anthropoid, android, and platypelloid. The anthropoid pelvis is usually seen in about 25% of women and could be challenging for vaginal births.

Ultimately, I found a physician 90 miles away and reached out for a consultation to determine if I qualified as a possible candidate for a VBAC. He requested my medical records from my previous cesarean sections and birth records, and we had an interview, including a physical examination to determine the shape of my pelvis. My doctor was older and wiser and definitely more experienced and less concerned about lawsuits. He had a level of confidence in his craft and the results he could produce, and his steady guidance helped to assuage my fears. Honestly, my doctor was God sent.

Thus, once I made the connection with him and determined that I qualified as a candidate for a VBAC, I began my appointments to prepare for the process. Securing my physician was just the first step in the process. While I got some relief in knowing that a part of the equation had been solved, I knew there was still a lot of work to do. The battle was only halfway won.

So, equipped with faith and knowing God was just a prayer away, I began to bring my request before God at each opportunity. I kept reminding him of his promises to me and my heart's desires. Taking my requests before God was a daily practice. Having to pray so often and believe for something that seemed impossible helped me to train my faith muscle. Almost daily, I had to fight the inner voice that tried to discourage me and instead stand on the truth of God's promises, reminding myself as often as I had to, that I would have a successful vaginal birth.

I went into the process knowing that I was crafted by a loving God, who took the time to remind me in His word that I am *"fearfully and wonderfully made"* (Psalm 139:14 KJV). I faced a good number of challenges, but my response each time was to go back to the word of God and find a scripture that spoke to each challenge I faced.

I had to borrow a page from how Jesus handled being tempted in the wilderness. At every juncture, He did not speak empty words to silence the devil but spoke back the word of God. If there's one promise God has given us about His word, it is that it always accomplishes its intended purposes. *"Faithful is He that calleth you, who also will do it"* (1 Thessalonians 5:24 KJV).

My path is indeed quite different and while I was able to have two consecutive vaginal births after having had two C-sections, I know the story is not the same for some women who approached the process with even greater awareness, the best medical team, and more robust faith. For those women, not being able to have a vaginal birth does not mean that they were somehow denied that experience by God, but just goes to show that God is all knowing and wiser than we are, and He determines the outcomes of lives in spite of our plans and best intentions. Ultimately, He knows why they were not able to go down that path and experience that journey and He redeems their pain and is providential in ways that will soothe their souls if they listen for His voice.

Ultimately, God's will was done in their lives, and the greatest blessing is still that sweet new baby scent and the eventual pitter-patter of little feet, a result which is still joyous irrespective of the method of birth.

As I navigated my desire to have a vaginal birth, reading through the New Testament and poring over the encounters Jesus had with a range of people, it is obvious he had a heart for women.

From the Samaritan woman to his friendship with the sister duo, Martha and Mary, to the woman with the issue of blood, his heart for women loomed large. With the woman who had been bleeding for years, her faith restored her back to health. However, it is obvious that Jesus had a desire for her body to function based on God's perfect design.

A case of bleeding that lasted over a decade clearly violates God's design and I wonder how disruptive that must have been to her fertility and ability to carry a baby. That Jesus would permit her healing shows that he desires normalcy even with our reproductive organs and I am so glad He extended His grace to me. While it was always my desire to give birth to all my children vaginally, I had my first two children via C-section.

In retrospect, while it was not what I wanted, I can appreciate the experience since it afforded me the lens through which to deeply connect with women who have had C-sections, as well as women who have had vaginal births, and those who have had C-sections but desire vaginal births. In the next chapter I will briefly describe my experience with both of my C-sections as they were quite instructive and honestly prepared me for my vaginal births.

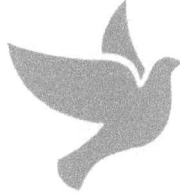

Chapter 2

Before VBAC, the Previous C-Sections

There is a time for everything, and a season for every activity under the heavens. —

Ecclesiastes 3:1 (NIV)

My first pregnancy was quite easy. I did not experience any morning sickness and there truly was nothing scary or out of the ordinary. Aside from the fact that I marveled at and was sometimes spooked by the idea of a living, breathing human growing inside me who would be born with ten fingers and ten toes, I had a relatively easy pregnancy.

I was still an emergency medicine resident then and was in the second year of my training. Interestingly, despite having gone through medical school and done rotations in obstetrics and gynecology, I had no clue what to expect with my own pregnancy.

Aside from a few people I knew from a distance who were pregnant and a handful of friends who had babies, all the information I had on what it meant to be pregnant was from medical school and gleaned from television shows and such.

Once I found out I was pregnant, I began the hunt for a good obstetrician. I read reviews online and also asked people who had used the doctors I was considering before I made the decision to entrust my pregnancy journey to the physician I chose. Also, I prayed about my decision and allowed God to guide me through the process. In the end, my doctor was fantastic! He had a great bedside manner and seemed to genuinely care about my pregnancy journey. I did not feel like a random statistic but felt that I mattered. My appointments were pretty routine: I would get my belly measured, provide urine and blood samples, have my blood pressure checked, my weight taken, and have the fetal heart tone of the baby checked, amongst other routine checks.

These visits occurred once a month in the early stage of my pregnancy. However, by the 28th week, I went more frequently. Mostly, there was nothing to ask on my part, or maybe I just did not know what to ask about as I was having a seemingly normal pregnancy.

Also, as I was going through the process, I thought I was a pro. As is common, I got congratulatory messages from people who were elated to see a baby carriage follow closely behind my wedding. Then came the advice and old wives' tales. I was advised to do squats. Some people recommended eating for two, advice which I found is totally inaccurate.

Others recommended a host of vitamins, and some suggested that I avoid working too much. Others tried to predict the baby's gender based on the shape of my belly, with some attributing heartburn to a baby with a head full of hair. Some were concerned with making sure I had a lot of sex, and others shared the utterly ridiculous notions that taking a bath could drown the baby and drinking lots of milk would ensure a copious supply of breastmilk. My pregnancy continued to progress normally, and at about my 39th week, I began having contractions and didn't know what to do.

Also, I was not quite sure what I was feeling. My legs and feet were swollen, and my blood pressure was elevated above what was the norm for me. With concerns of preeclampsia looming, I had to be admitted to the hospital, starting the journey of having my baby.

As fate would have it, the obstetrician who had been seeing me and was familiar with my medical history went on vacation at about the same time. As my blood pressure numbers continued to rise, the attending physician on call who was caring for me got worried about the risk of preeclampsia and decided that labor should be induced. As a first-time mom and a doctor, I had some idea, but I did not quite understand the process. Induction before delivery is the process of using either medication or tools to start the process of labor. Once I got assigned a room, the doctor came in and broke my water. From the moment your water is broken, you are being timed and you are not allowed to labor for more than 12 to 24 hours because of the risk of infections. Because I was a primigravida[5] mom, there usually is little delay because the body is not used to the labor and delivery process; hence

---

[5] A woman who is pregnant for the first time.

the chances of having a cesarean section are high if active labor does not progress.

I started the process at 7:00 in the morning, and at that time, I was lying still in bed, with little to no movement and no repositioning. I was also given an epidural. In retrospect, I realize that the lack of movement and the early administration of an epidural were all factors that worked against a vaginal delivery.

I was makeup ready and was just waiting for the baby to make his grand appearance and take pictures, but it seemed like little was happening to get me to the point of delivering my baby. Twelve hours later, almost an entire half-day since the process of labor began, the doctor came in and advised that a cesarean section would be necessary. The thought of a cesarean section was disappointing, and I remember crying, as that was not what I wanted. If I had done more research and had been more knowledgeable about the birth process, I would have been in a better position to advocate for myself, but as a first-time mom, if clueless was a person, it surely was me!

So, what does a cesarean section feel like? If you have spent some time watching any medical shows that involve the birth of a child, you've likely seen the procedure dramatized, but might still have questions about what actually occurs.

A cesarean section is the surgical delivery of a baby through a cut or incision made in the mother's abdomen and uterus. Health care providers use it when they believe it is safer for the mother, baby, or both.

Once I began the process of labor, I was given an epidural. Epidurals are often talked about, but if you have not experienced the process of labor, understanding how the epidural delivery process works might be a bit of a mystery. It need not be. Epidurals are administered via the back vertebrae, through a procedure that is just like a lumbar puncture. The purpose is to stop pain in some parts of the body. Epidurals are injected into the epidural space, versus being administered into the dural sac (with a spinal anesthesia), which provides immediate relief.

Spinal anesthesia is preferred by some because the baby is exposed to a lower amount of medication; however, both methods have the same end goal.

The process of administering the epidural took about five minutes from start to finish and I was fully awake. While I was given an epidural, it is not uncommon for general anesthesia to be administered if needed.

During a cesarean section, only one family member is usually allowed into the operating room to prevent overcrowding. In my case, my husband was allowed to come in and was at the head of the bed and did cut the umbilical cord. I could see the baby through the blue surgical drapes and, to be honest, the process felt quite sterile. In retrospect, there are some things I would have done differently to make the process feel more personal and less mechanical, such as having a birth plan that stated my needs. I'm convinced that having a birth plan and a doula is important so you can specify what you want, because oftentimes the baby is taken away and all a new mom gets is just a glimpse of her new infant being carted away as the infant wails. With a vaginal birth, you get your baby at once for skin-to-skin bonding. More recently, skin-to-skin bonding is now offered with cesarean sections.

Cesarean sections are major surgeries, and anytime there is a major surgery, scar tissue is created.

There are several complications that can occur during the process and several years afterwards. Adhesions can occur later in the future, which could lead to bowel obstructions and adhesion pains. There are also complications that can arise from vaginal births, so this is not to say one is better than the other.

When my first baby was 17 months old, I conceived again. As with the first baby, my second was also unplanned as well. However, by the time I conceived the second baby, I was done with my residency program. At this point, I was aware that a vaginal birth was possible even after a caesarean section, and I wanted to give that option a try. So, I started looking for a doctor who could do a VBAC. Again, it was an easy pregnancy, and the baby was properly positioned. However, at 39 weeks, the baby moved and got repositioned. Instead of his head being down, the baby was now in a transverse position. This means the baby was lying horizontally across the uterus, rather than being vertical.

At that point, it was determined that I could labor on my own and have a vaginal birth if only the baby would reposition himself. So, my doctor allowed me to progress to 41 weeks to see if the baby would naturally be repositioned.

When I went for my appointment after that time had elapsed, the baby was still transverse. Again, I was clueless and did not do as much research to see if it was possible to get the baby repositioned. I was not aware that I could find a doctor who would be committed to assisting with repositioning the baby.

Also, I came to find out that for some women facing this same challenge, some doctors would give the assurance of repositioning the baby but would not follow through. Thus, since the baby was still transverse at 41 weeks, my doctor determined that another cesarean section would be necessary. I became quite tearful as I was with my first baby, and I didn't want to follow through with future appointments. I had to ultimately have a cesarean section to deliver my baby.

Unlike my first cesarean section, my surgery was scheduled and was much better the second time around. It was quicker and faster, as I was in and out with minimal time being wasted. With my second cesarean section, I was given spinal anesthesia, which differed from the epidural I was given the first time. What makes spinal anesthesia different from an epidural? A spinal anesthesia is a one-time dose.

With my second cesarean section, the recovery process was much better. It seemed as though I was becoming a cesarean section pro, but I didn't want that badge. I still kept on nursing my desire to have a vaginal birth and hoped that the next time I had a baby I would get my opportunity. I knew that having a vaginal birth after a cesarean section would be an uphill climb, not just physically, but mentally too.

In spite of the challenge that loomed, I was not deterred and figured I would attempt a try and see how far my faith and sheer resolve would carry me.

Thus, I began a journey to understand the process of having a VBAC and began to prepare to have my next baby vaginally. To be honest, I did not expect the process to be a cakewalk, and as I began to expand my research and gather information, I realized that having a vaginal birth after two cesarean sections would require a holistic and honest evaluation that would then lead to diligent planning in order to achieve my goal. Ultimately, my introspection reaffirmed my decision. In the next chapter, I will share the steps I took to prepare for a vaginal delivery after having had two cesarean sections.

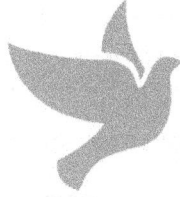

CHAPTER 3

PREPARING FOR YOUR VBAC

For which of you, desiring to build a tower, does not first sit down and count the cost, whether he has enough to complete it? — Luke 14:28 (ESV)

From the moment you decide you want to have a VBAC with a future pregnancy, you need to start planning. The American College of Obstetricians and Gynecologists (ACOG) advises a waiting period of 18 months after having a cesarean before attempting a VBAC to avoid complications.

A waiting period is advisable because this time allows for healing, formulating an exercise routine, and getting on track with a proper diet, all factors which have been known to affect the outcome of a VBAC attempt. Another recommendation is to join a VBAC community, to aid in the process of gathering critical information to guarantee success.

Most cities have groups on social media, and it is usually advisable to join because knowledge is power. The groups provide support and information on doctors and hospitals and other care specialists. Overall, an important factor to consider is information acquisition to become somewhat of an expert as this will help build your confidence and enable you to be a better advocate for yourself.

Get Your Body Ready

Preparing for a VBAC involves teaching your body a new birth narrative. Since your body experienced a cesarean section as its first foray into birthing, your body needs to be retrained to learn a new form of birthing. You have to challenge old notions of what you think your body and mind are capable of doing. Thus, give your body time to heal before attempting a VBAC.

Be honest and sincere with yourself. Be at peace with your previous birth story while you hope for a successful VBAC. I took four years to allow my body to heal between my last caesarean section and first vaginal birth.

Start with Self-assessment

The biggest question you might need to ask yourself before diving into the process is why you want a vaginal birth. Vaginal births are God's design because the process fully utilizes the birth canal and is the perfect design for bringing babies into the world. Because a vaginal birth is the body's proper channel for birth, there are a host of benefits, including quicker recovery time and lower chances for complications for future pregnancies.

Granted, for any medical procedures or birthing methods in general, there are complications that can occur, and you should acquaint yourself with the complications that could result from either a vaginal delivery or a cesarean section. Pondering the complications that could arise from either can bring along feelings of fear and anxiety to our minds, but we need to remember to not be afraid even as we do our due diligence in gaining the necessary knowledge.

Remember, *"For God hath not given us the spirit of fear; but of power, and of love, and of a sound mind"* (2 Timothy 1:7 KJV).

The benefits of a vaginal birth are quite numerous, but after having had a caesarean section, the importance of a thorough mental evaluation and an honest discussion with yourself, your community, and your medical provider about your reasons for wanting to attempt a vaginal birth cannot be overstated. However, before you involve your community or provider, you need to know your why and this varies for every woman. Whatever your reasons are, they are valid. I mention knowing your why because as you journey towards a vaginal delivery process, you might be discouraged and decide to go through with what is your usual, a caesarean section. However, knowing your why will keep you on track and will help you continue to forge ahead.

Depending on when you had your caesarean section, you want to ensure that your body has had enough time to heal before embarking on another pregnancy journey. When thinking of your body, pay attention to the scars and ensure that you are fully healed and do not feel any discomfort.

Your uterus also needs time to heal as it has had to stretch to accommodate a pregnancy, endured an incision, and self-healed. The passage of time has to be trusted to have done its work to heal your body as it best can; however, you still need to proceed with caution. You know your body best and more than any assessment from a professional to steer you in any direction, you intuitively know with some guidance what your body is capable of enduring. Trust signals and cues from your body and do not push your body beyond its limits. Our bodies are well-built machines that can withstand so much, but you need to make sure that your body aligns with signals from your mind as the two are inextricably linked. If you do not feel as though your body and mind might be in sync, that might be a cue to reevaluate your plan and rethink a different strategy. Also, it is okay to give yourself a break or even decide to go through with another cesarean section if you are not fully prepared to go all in on a vaginal birth.

Prepare Your Mind

When it comes to pregnancy and delivery, it is important to acknowledge that God is in control, and while you may not be able to control the outcome or type of delivery, you can still hope for a certain kind of experience.

Knowing this, be prepared for an outcome that may be other than what you desire; however, trust that how your birth journey ends is by God's design and is perfect for you.

When I began hoping for a vaginal birth, one of my prayers was, "Father, I pray that there will be no emergent reason to be rushed for an emergency cesarean section." I kept praying about this occurrence because it is not uncommon to plan for a vaginal birth and then end up having a caesarean section.

Preparing your mind involves teaching your body to respond to certain mental cues. A lot starts in the mind and oftentimes battles are won or lost in our minds. Our minds are great repositories, helping us use experience to move through mental maps that we have created over time to help us survive. There are many ways to get your mind ready and to essentially convince it that it can actually birth a baby, without scars. Meditation, self-affirmation, deep breathing, deep relaxation, and other practices can be helpful in retraining the mind.

No matter what the outcome of your birth story, resist the urge to see your story as a failure, because you are an amazing woman who just performed something that truly is miraculous and one who loves her child dearly.

Process Previous Cesarean Sections

Evaluate each previous cesarean section experience, cataloging what went well and what went wrong. Even though a c-section might not have been what you preferred, take the time to evaluate the experience in its entirety, noting what was unpleasant and what you believe went well with the experience. If you had to go through a caesarean section again, what aspects of the experience would you improve on and what would you totally nix out of the mix? If you had a traumatic birthing experience, consider reaching out to a licensed therapist to help process the experience, as it might be a bit challenging to parse through your feelings on your own without a fresh lens and a trained voice.

Also, talk about the experience with trusted friends or loved ones who can guarantee a judgment-free zone to enable you to freely share the full gamut of the experience and who are supportive of your decision to experience a vaginal birth.

Additionally, spend some time learning about what types of medical treatments you received and why such options were presented.

Some items to consider are what kind of incision was performed. Usually, if it was not an emergency C-section, it was most likely a transverse incision, meaning you can have a VBAC with reduced risks for uterine rupture. If it was an emergency C-section, in most cases, the incision likely would have been vertical, and this poses risks for uterine rupture and could reduce your chances for future pregnancies. Other checklist items to consider are what kind of pain management methods were employed and if you were induced, as the chances for a caesarean section are higher with inductions when labor has not actively started. Also, obtain medical records from your previous cesarean sections and take these along to your first doctor's visit.

Do Your Research

It's vital that you do your research. There are so many resources at your fingertips, you should maximize and use them fully. However, in a sea of so much information, verify every source and when in doubt, talk to a trusted and knowledgeable medical practitioner who is acquainted with your plans and the goal you would like to achieve.

Do not neglect to do your homework. Read as much as you can about the VBAC process. Knowledge is power and ignorance cannot be an excuse as you pursue this goal. There are many books, including mine, as well as scientific data and publications that can provide useful insights and guidance. Reading stories from other women regarding how they achieved a successful VBAC can be both instructive and inspiring. I did a lot of reading and internet searches and literally turned over many tables in search of the information I needed.

YouTube videos can be educational as well as provide some positive reinforcement and even visuals that are easy to understand. However, with YouTube videos, be especially mindful about the content you choose to watch and make sure the videos you choose are created and posted by reputable and reliable organizations. Being able to watch and rewatch certain videos is helpful in creating a visual image that creates a new mental framework. I watched a lot of positive YouTube videos on vaginal births and the stories made a difference in shaping my mind positively. Learn about fetal positioning and watch videos on prenatal classes.

Pain Relief

You also want to learn about non-medicated methods and ways to reduce pain during labor. Some ways of reducing pain during labor without using medications include certain tailored movements, using birthing balls, asking your partner or doula to us acupuncture points to relieve pain, deep relaxation, and water birthing.

With my first baby, I was induced, got IV fluids, was in bed and not moving around, hardly changing position. In retrospect, I learned that the fluids I got and the immobility worked against labor and were a factor in slowing down my progression of labor.

In terms of pain management during delivery, the use of epidurals is often hotly debated. However, based on my personal experience, I believe epidurals might have slowed down the progression of labor for me. However, if you must, you can have an epidural as every woman responds differently. With my vaginal births, I did not receive an epidural and so I had to find ways to relax and recenter to focus my mind on having a vaginal birth.

With one of my vaginal births, I wanted to power through and avoid getting an epidural, but as labor progressed, the pain was so intense that I was literally begging the medical personnel to give me an epidural. My doctor, however, kept encouraging me to persevere and just soldier on, and I am glad he did because shortly after the episode of intense pain, my baby was delivered. I share this to let you know that you can surely show yourself some grace, and if you feel you want to end the process at any time and opt to receive an epidural, do not hold back. Do what you feel is best for you. Your mothering skills are not predicated on how you birthed your baby.

VBAC Risk Score

Prior to deciding to attempt a VBAC, it is useful to use a VBAC scoring system to predict your likelihood of a successful VBAC attempt. The calculations include age, height, weight, reason for previous cesarean deliveries, and whether a person was being treated for high blood pressure, amongst other factors.

Previously, race was used as a factor, but most calculations have removed it, since women who identified as Black or

Hispanic typically received a lower score than counterparts who identified as White. Typically, a higher VBAC score suggests a greater chance that a vaginal birth will be successful.

Exercise and Diet

Exercise regularly and eat well. There are many exercise routines and dieting plans that are quite useful, and it is advisable to seek out an exercise routine that gives you good results and works with your lifestyle. Another helpful tip is to evaluate your weight and be willing to lose a few pounds before conception. I lost 30 pounds to get my body ready for the process. Along with regular exercise. balanced nutrition helps you to maintain physical and mental stamina. Drink lots of water and avoid caffeinated drinks. Also, consider taking vitamins, supplements, and herbs that may help strengthen the uterine wall. These include raspberry leaf tea and evening primrose oil, which helps with cervical dilation. Find ways to relax and explore options that are helpful in reducing stress. Work on learning ways to relax your entire body, especially when you are in pain.

Create a Birth Plan

Your birth plan is in many ways your birthing constitution and your core team members need a copy. A birth plan is a document that lets your medical team know your labor and delivery preferences in regard to things like pain management, postpartum care, newborn procedures, and even the ambience in the room. Your partner, the doula, doctor, nurses, and the person transporting you to the hospital all need to have a copy handed to them ahead of time. Have it in your file as part of the documents you intend to take to the hospital and make extra copies. Also, consider leaving copies ahead of time in the car you hope might take you to the hospital when you do go into labor. If possible, save a digital copy on your electronic devices as well. Importantly, schedule time to sit down with your doctor to go over the plan so that he or she has visibility and knowledge about what your wishes are. There are a good number of birth plans that can be found online by doing a search on the internet. The Bump has a good birth plan template; however, there are others that might be more suited for your needs.[6]

[6] "What Is a Birth Plan and Why Is It Important?" The Bump Editors, medically reviewed by Kendra Segura, MD, Updated October 19, 2023, https://www.thebump.com/a/tool-birth-plan

Importantly, prepare for the possibility of another cesarean section. With most hospitals and doctors, including those that are VBAC friendly, you will be required to sign a consent for a cesarean section as a backup plan just in case trial of labor after C-section (TOLAC) fails. It is okay to prepare your mind for a possible caesarean section and have a backup plan so as not to be disappointed and taken by surprise.

In the event that you do have a caesarean section, explore your options for a family-centered cesarean section which allows for skin-to-skin contact after birth, breastfeeding in the operating room, using transparent drapes or lowering of the drapes so you can see the baby during delivery and other options that can help create an environment that feels less like a medicated birth and more like a vaginal delivery.

Build Your Community

Curate your community carefully. The first members of your community usually are the team of people you have purposefully built around you. But beyond your core team, you are going to have to build out a community of people with shared experiences to journey with.

Just like choosing your team begins long before you perhaps even decide to try for another baby and birth narrative, your community should also be built out way ahead of time.

Seek out community locally either by asking your medical team or by simply doing some research. There are several communities on social media and other online forums that are quite helpful. Your main goal is finding the necessary support to help you prevent an unnecessary caesarean section. Be committed to searching for a local group or subgroup that will provide this. With most online or Facebook groups, you are often vetted before being allowed to join the group. These groups contain a wealth of information and should be used as a tool.

When curating your community, be very strategic. Choose and join groups that resonate with your personal ideals. Make a list of your core values, your intentions for wanting to experience a vaginal birth, and weigh in your temperament as well, as online communities and social media can be unforgiving spaces. Know what your mental threshold truly is. Think of your community in terms that make sense to you. You could liken it to putting together an art show, preparing a dish, or maybe even conducting an orchestra.

All the different elements have to work well together. As different as the support groups might be, there has to be harmony between all parts. Again, do not hesitate to withdraw from a community that does not seem like a good fit or one that does not seem to steer you toward your goal. You owe it to yourself to be the architect of your own desire.

Prepare Your Team

Your team should be made up of people you can honestly trust to advocate for you should you for any reason be unable to speak for yourself. These people should be well acquainted with your birth plan and know it just as well as you do. You should start putting your team together once you decide to have a vaginal birth. Your team might grow or dwindle over time and that is fine. You should feel comfortable enough with the people on your team and be vulnerable with them as well. Your team should include your chosen village. In many cases, the roster will include your spouse, close family, your doctor, nurses, a midwife or a doula, and importantly, a therapist or someone you can be truly vulnerable with in candid conversation.

Your team will have to rally around you and cheer you on every step of the way. You will have to Be honest with them about your emotions and the reasons for your desire for a VBAC. They will be your biggest cheerleaders. Thus, in a sense you also have a twofold job. While you get yourself ready, you need to bring your team along and get them ready too. You're all batting for the same larger team in a sense and the success of your VBAC will largely depend on selecting a team that is supportive, understands your goal, and is just as committed as you are to its actualization.

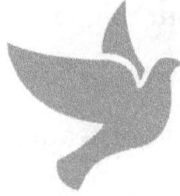

CHAPTER 4

GET YOUR TEAM READY

Two are better than one, because they have a good reward for their labor. For if they fall, one will lift up his companion. But woe to him that is alone when he falls, for he has no one to help him up. —
Ecclesiastes 4:9-10 *(NIV)*

While raising children, it is not uncommon to hear the popular African adage, "it takes a village." Oftentimes, it is said in consolation to a new mother struggling to juggle motherhood and still find some balance, to let her know that she is not alone on her mothering journey.

It is meant to assure her that there is a community waiting in the wings, ready to step in and offer support to the mother and the children, and provide help where needed, as the task of childrearing should not just be left to the nuclear family. While I prepared to have my babies, I often wondered how much different the process would be if members of the village were present long before the baby's birth.

Having a baby is quite personal, but it is also communal. Some cultures have traditions such as baby showers and extensive mentoring from older women as an expectant mom prepares to nest, but in some instances, the pregnancy journey can be a lonely road. Some mothers manage their changing bodies and prepare for what might be one of the biggest events in their life all by themselves. I pondered upon how an expanded concept of the village that begins at conception would be such a game changer for most women, and especially for women such as myself, planning to take on a VBAC challenge. Luckily, I was able to curate an exceptional team that was supportive of my desire for a VBAC, that took the time to understand my needs including becoming familiar with my birth plan, and that championed me all the way to my desired goal.

Thus, the importance of a village cannot be overstated. The village should include not just your partner and immediate family, but support groups and providers. In a sense, you have to raise your village so they can in turn raise your child.

A reasonable first step is to get your partner on board and make sure they're supportive of your plans. You are both in this together and ideally, your partner should be your biggest advocate and cheerleader. Deciding to have a vaginal delivery after a cesarean section is a major feat and you want to ensure that you are fully supported. There might be days when you want to opt for a cesarean section because it is familiar and because frankly, the thought of a vaginal birth might be daunting. You want to make sure your partner understands your desire to have a vaginal birth and the reasons for your choice.

Having seen you undergo a previous cesarean section, your partner is fully acquainted with the time it took you to recover after having the baby and the physical and emotional toll the process took on your body. The recovery time does impact the care you are able to provide for your children and family soon after the delivery and nursing may be impacted, especially since a scar has to be managed as it fully heals.

Your family's budget and financial goals are also impacted, as cesarean sections and the resulting hospital stays are longer and more expensive than for a vaginal birth. Also, the longer recovery time impacts and delays sexual intimacy after birth.

While most providers recommend a waiting period of two to six weeks to resume sexual activity regardless of the delivery method, with a cesarean section the wait time might be a bit longer to give the incision time to fully heal. Given all these reasons, it is quite evident that the decision to have a vaginal birth after a cesarean section is a team sport and not a solo effort. Assuming you and your spouse have decided that you would like to attempt a vaginal birth, bringing them onboard means acquainting them with all the plans. Your partner should know your why and also be able to articulate the birth plan just as well as you can. Obviously, the physical experiences are yours, but you would want your partner to be emotionally invested as well.

Having your partner be your team member looks like them knowing every detail of your plans and getting acquainted with the terminology and the process. If your partner is a deep empath, they will feel all the emotions and experience all that comes with the process — except the physical aspects.

Does your partner know what your birth plan looks like, is your partner able to articulate your needs to your provider, is your partner able to advocate on your behalf, ask the necessary questions, and ensure you get the results you desire? When you are deep in the throes of the labor process, is your partner able to be a sentinel and still steer the boat safely to the harbor? Having a disinterested partner can impede your process and desire for a vaginal birth because you will need a lot of support; that's why your partner needs to buy into your desire and be supportive. Once you are sure you have the support of your partner, hand them a whistle — you have just signed up the first member of your team.

If for some reason you have a spouse who is disinterested and unwilling to support your desire to have a vaginal birth, find ways to navigate this hurdle and look for other people who will encourage you and provide the necessary support. However, it is important to get your partner's support, as you will need it when the rubber meets the road. Also, because you are a team, give consideration to your partner as well and allow them to feel heard. For example, a friend wanted a VBAC but did not have her husband's support and so decided against it. He was concerned about uterine rupture and so, as a team, they eventually opted for a cesarian section.

Join a Support Group

Connect with your local International Cesarean Awareness Network (ICAN) group. You could also join a VBAC community on Facebook and a local ICAN group in your community. I joined a local Facebook group. The reason for this suggestion is the local groups provide a wealth of information on VBAC-friendly communities and doctors. Your local ICAN group is a good place to start on your VBAC journey, just as I did. I just did a Google search and that is how I became aware of ICAN and the wealth of resources that were available. In our digital age, there is so much information at our fingertips and we need to take advantage of it. I looked for a local ICAN group but did not find one close by, so I joined a group in the nearest big metropolis. A big benefit in joining a support group was being able to use the group to vet providers. Through my group affiliation,

I got a list of providers that were recommended and those that were not recommended. Because my research for care providers showed that there were no VBAC-friendly doctors where I lived, I had to commit to making the drive to the nearest big city.

Interview Your Providers

Find a VBAC-friendly doctor and research the hospitals where the provider has admitting privileges. Do not use a doctor who is VBAC friendly but does not have the required privileges. Usually, VBAC-friendly hospitals have anesthesiologists present on call 24/7, as this is one of the requirements for hospitals to be VBAC friendly. Keep in mind that tertiary centers like teaching hospitals and major institutional hospitals are preferable to community hospitals when it comes to finding a VBAC-friendly facility.

Find a few providers — physicians and nurses — and meet with them. Do not hold back on questions. Ask broadly. If any question crosses your mind, that means you need to bring it up. Check cesarean section rates and VBAC success rates. Make it clear that having a VBAC is your desired outcome. Some doctors might say they are VBAC friendly but not follow through. Make sure any doctor taking calls for your provider is VBAC friendly in the event that circumstances lead to your regular provider not being available when you do go into labor. You can find out more about hospital policies on their website and what restrictions or limitations they are subject to.

Expand Your Team

Your team should include more than physicians and nurses. Doulas, midwives, and childbirth educators are usually quite experienced and should form a core part of your team. I was a bit skeptical about the need for a doula but once I engaged the services of one, I became a fierce advocate for using their services. I would highly recommend the use of a doula even for women who might choose to have elective cesarean sections. My doula was quite helpful and came to one of my doctor's appointments. She had a copy of my birth plan and was supportive throughout the entire process. Some doulas will even provide postpartum care, which is extremely invaluable.

For the birth of my youngest child, my doctor made an exception that permitted my doula to be present even though there were Covid-19 restrictions that only allowed a spouse to be present for the birth. Thus, be sure to ask about restrictions, ask about hospital policies for VBAC, ask doctors about their partners and those who cover for them. Importantly, find and hire a doula experienced in VBACs and with sufficient knowledge to help with optimal positioning of the baby for safe vaginal delivery.

Let's take a closer look at the roles played by doulas, midwives, and childbirth educators.

Doulas

A doula is a woman, typically without obstetric training, who is employed to provide guidance and support to a pregnant woman during labor. A doula provides both emotional and physical support before, during, and after a woman's pregnancy and especially during childbirth. While doulas receive some form of training, they are not medical professionals and should not replace trained personnel. They also do not deliver babies or provide medical assistance and care. Their primary role is to serve as advocates during the pregnancy journey and sometimes beyond.

Doulas can be hired to provide assistance during labor and birth. Some doulas provide antepartum support for women who are put on bedrest to prevent preterm labor, and others are postpartum doulas that offer support for the new mother during the first weeks after birth. Some services offered by a doula, most of which begin in the second or third trimester, will include teaching the mother relaxation and breathing skills helping to develop a birth plan, answering questions about the birth process, and getting the mother ready to care for her new baby.

During labor, the role of the doula is to provide support and comfort as labor progresses. The doula does this by helping the mother get into comfortable positions, ensuring that the mother has adequate fluids and nutrition, providing massages to help the mother relax, as well as by being a liaison and communicating the mother's preferences to the medical team. After labor, the doula provides support as the mother transitions to the home and teaches her how to care for the baby and herself. Doulas may also assist with breastfeeding education, coach other family members in providing the best care for the mom, and ensure that rest and proper nutrition are not neglected as the mother tends to her new baby.

Midwives

Midwives are trained nurses who specialize in women's reproductive health and childbirth. They receive training that enables them to oversee low-risk pregnancies, labor, and birth.

Midwives also have expanded services that include other obstetric and gynecological services such as performing pelvic exams. Further, they are trained to care for women from adolescence through the menopausal years. Midwives perform similar roles to obstetricians and gynecologists but focus on natural techniques for childbirth and reproductive care. The scope of practice of a midwife includes confirming and dating pregnancy, providing prenatal and postpartum care, educating new mothers on infant care, supporting with breastfeeding, performing preventive health screenings and tests, and diagnosing and treating gynecological disorders such as sexually transmitted diseases and infertility.

Childbirth Educators

Childbirth educators are experts in the development and delivery of educational resources surrounding labor and birth. They are not clinicians and do not have medial training but rather get certified to function in their roles. Some educators are advocates of the natural process of birth and teach expectant mothers to make informed decisions while educating them about other alternatives.

Decide on Your Facility

An essential part of your team is the providers at the facility you choose. Whether you choose to have a home birth, a hospital-based birth, or use a birthing center, the providers at the facility and their wealth of knowledge will be an invaluable resource.

My initial choice for a VBAC was a home birth. I had already experienced two hospital births and was not quite keen on a birthing center. I was wary of having a hospital birth because I did not want to end up having another cesarean section that involved being overly medicated with minimal control over the process. However, the midwife I found was not keen on a home birth and was not willing to accept me as a patient because I had had two previous C-sections. I had to then reevaluate my options and choose a hospital since it offered more control and better checks in place if any complications arose.

Often, home births are discouraged for women who have had more than one cesarean section. Most midwives have intervention plans in place in case of emergencies. However, you need to ask a series of questions to understand what arrangements they have with a hospital ahead of time.

If the birthing facility or midwife does not have a plan with a hospital, engaging an EMS service that is aware of the situation beforehand is often advisable. Many midwives who perform home births have a doctor on call they can engage. Let's look at the pros and cons of each.

Home Birth

Before engaging a midwife for a home birth, inquire about how many deliveries, complications, transfers to hospitals, and other challenges the midwife may have encountered. While broaching the topic might be a bit uncomfortable, the number of mortalities, if any, is important to note as well as emergency plans they have in place in the event things go awry. Because pregnancy and delivery are so unpredictable, life-threatening problems can occur during labor and delivery, so it is essential to discuss contingency plans with your certified midwife and have an arrangement in place for emergencies if you opt for a home birth. Research and statistics show that home-based births are associated with higher risks of infant mortality.

Birthing at home is void of effective fetal monitoring, and congenital or genetic diseases that may be discovered at birth in a hospital may be missed with a home birth.

Pros of a home birth:

1. Give birth in the comfort of your home.
2. A home birth allows for the avoidance of unnecessary medical interventions.
3. You have greater control over the birthing experience.

Cons of a home birth:

1. Home births are not safe for everyone and should only be attempted after individual risk factors have been evaluated.
2. In some cases, insurance does not cover home births.
3. Patients seeking to avoid being in a hospital might still end up being transferred to one in the case of an emergency.

Birthing Centers

Birthing centers are quite different from hospitals. Birthing centers are designed to deliver holistic care and provide a nurturing environment with comprehensive midwifery care.

The process is designed to be comfortable and involves less medical intervention. With these centers, proximity to a hospital that can provide around-the-clock maternity care is quite key in the event that complications do arise during the birthing process.

Pros of a birthing center:
1. Less medical interventions such as pain medication, labor induction, fetal heart rate monitoring, pelvic checks or delivery assisted with forceps or other instruments are at a minimum.
2. You have better control of the birthing process
3. Less expensive when compared to hospital birth

Cons of a birthing center:
1. Cultural or religious concerns
2. Access to transportation may not be available

Signs It's Time to Head to the Hospital
Sometimes complications arise during a home birth or at a birthing center. Here's when you may want to head for the hospital.

(This list is not all-inclusive; other circumstances may arise that also merit a trip to the hospital, so please listen to your team.)

1. Labor is delayed and not progressing
2. Signs of fetal distress
3. Fetal positioning is not conducive for vaginal delivery
4. Unbearable pain
5. Elevated blood pressure
6. Vaginal bleeding
7. Fever

Hospital Birth

Most births in the developed world are usually in hospitals and offer certain advantages that are not associated with other birthing facilities. One of the benefits of a hospital birth is access to pain medication including epidurals. Other benefits of birthing a baby in a hospital include having a plethora of medical personnel and a wealth of experienced support staff. Additionally, in the event that there are fetal complications, being in a hospital provides access to a neonatal intensive care unit (NICU) if the baby happens to be in distress post birth, where each second is precious and could be life altering for the infant.

Pros of a hospital:

1. Hospitals are better able to manage pain and have better pain prevention methods.

2. Hospitals have knowledgeable support staff with several years of experience.

3. Hospitals have access to neonatal intensive care units that could provide lifesaving options for your baby.

Cons of a hospital:

1. You have less control over the birthing process as the doctor might ultimately opt for the method that will deliver the best outcome.

2. There is the possibility that you might be seen by a doctor other than the one who attended to you throughout your pregnancy.

3. You will only be allowed to attempt a limited range of birthing positions in the hospital.

4. Also, once you're in labor, you are not allowed to have anything by mouth. This may sometimes be modified, depending on your physician, to allow only clear liquids by mouth.

As you continue to prepare for your VBAC, you will come to appreciate the value of a carefully selected team.

From having a supportive partner who is willing to cheer you on and help boost your morale on days when you would rather not bother with attempting a VBAC, to support groups that share stories of resilience and triumph to help encourage you, balanced by acknowledging their failed attempts to help you be measured in your approach, to a doula with years of experience, and the comfort of a facility that suits your needs, your team is the village you always needed but just had to create.

Ultimately, the hope is that a supportive team will free up your time to focus on other important aspects of your journey, like providing proper nourishment for your growing "baby bump."

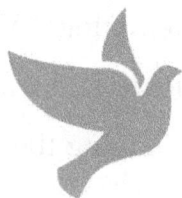

CHAPTER 5

CHOOSE A HEALTHY DIET FOR
PROPER NUTRITION

But Daniel resolved that he would not defile himself with the king's food, or with the wine that he drank. Therefore, he asked the chief of the eunuchs to allow him not to defile himself. And God gave Daniel favor and compassion in the sight of the chief and the eunuchs. — Daniel 1:8,9 (ESV)

Preparing for a baby requires making some changes, often including a major adjustment of your dietary intake. To maintain a healthy pregnancy, you will need to increase your daily caloric intake by about 300 extra calories consisting of fruits, vegetables, proteins, and whole grains. You'll also need to reduce your consumption of excessive sweets and fats. A healthy diet during pregnancy is necessary to keep you and the baby nourished and also can be helpful in alleviating some pregnancy symptoms such as nausea and constipation.

Along with being mindful of the types of food you ingest while you are expecting, another important part of your diet that needs to be adjusted is your fluid intake. The recommendation for fluid intake during pregnancy is several glasses of water in addition to other fluid sources like soups, fruits, and juices. Some fluids, like coffee or tea containing caffeine, will need to be regulated, and in some instances, eliminated altogether. If you drink caffeinated beverages often, consider speaking with the health care providers managing your pregnancy for advice on how best to proceed. Importantly, avoid alcohol entirely. Proper hydration during pregnancy is necessary as dehydration can often have some adverse consequences, including preterm labor and abnormal contractions.

Nutrition During Pregnancy

A good balanced diet and proper nutrition during pregnancy are essential and play a big role in your pregnancy and delivery outcomes. There is a common myth that a pregnant woman with cravings needs to overindulge since she is essentially eating for two.

However, giving in to every impulse and eating without restraint can lead to excessive weight gain that may further lead to complications in pregnancy like gestational diabetes, preeclampsia, preterm birth, birth injury, a large baby, and quite possibly a cesarean section. Pregnant women on average should only increase their caloric intake by 340 extra calories in their second and third trimester if pregnant with a single baby; When pregnant with twins, an expectant mom will need to increase her caloric intake by 600, and by 900 if pregnant with triplets, based on recommendations from the American College of Obstetricians and Gynecologists.

Plan Healthy Meals

It is essential to follow a healthy eating routine while pregnant. Your meals should contain healthy foods you enjoy.

In planning your meals, include fruits, vegetables, whole grains, low-fat or fat-free dairy, oils, and proteins. In between meals, opt for healthy snacks. If you have bouts of nausea, healthy options like dry whole grain cereal, toast, and saltines are good remedies. Below is a list of some food suggestions to help build your meal kit:

- Grains (include a healthy serving of whole grains)
- Bread
- Pasta
- Oatmeal
- Fruits
- Vegetables
- Protein
- Dairy

A resource I found helpful while creating meals is the MyPlate website, created by the US Department of Agriculture. MyPlate recommends five food groups: fruits, grains, vegetables, proteins, and dairy. The MyPlate website, **www.myplate.gov**, can guide you in making healthy food choices.

Take Your Prenatal Vitamins

While a healthy diet is important during pregnancy, supplements are necessary to provide vitamins and minerals that you need. Most of these supplements are necessary not just when you are pregnant but are also necessary while you're trying to conceive. Prenatal vitamins are quite important as you need greater quantities of certain vitamins while pregnant or trying to conceive.

For example, taking folic acid prenatally is necessary to prevent neural tube defects, which are serious abnormalities of the fetal brain and spinal cord. Another necessary supplement is iron, which helps your body make blood to supply oxygen to the fetus and prevent anemia. While it is important to increase the intake of certain supplements, always check with your health care provider to ensure that you are taking the right supplements, as excess intake of certain supplements might be harmful to the growing fetus.

Key Vitamins Needed during Pregnancy
- Calcium for bone health
- Choline for healthy fetal brain and spinal cord development
- Folic acid for the prevention of neural tube defects

- Iodine for brain development
- Iron for red blood cell growth and oxygen delivery to the fetus
- Vitamin A for healthy skin and eyes and for bone growth (do not take in excess as it could be teratogenic and result in birth defects)
- Vitamin B6/Vitamin B12 helps form red blood cells and maintains the nervous system
- Vitamin C for healthy gums, teeth, and bones
- Vitamin D for strong bones

Herbs for VBAC Preparation

For many centuries, childbearing women have employed the use of herbs to help with pregnancy, labor, and delivery. In different communities, midwives have depended on different herbs and there are a few that have become quite popular. The evidence supporting the use of some, for example, raspberry leaves, still needs further research to address the effectiveness of the herb, despite its popularity.[7]

---

[7] Rebekah Bowman, Jan Taylor, Sally Muggleton, and Deborah Davis, "Biophysical Effects, Safety and Efficacy of Raspberry Leaf Use in Pregnancy: A Systematic Integrative Review," *BMC Complementary Medicine and Therapies*, Vol. 21, February 9, 2021, **https://www.ncbi.nlm.nih.gov/pmc/articles/PMC7871383/**

You should consult with your physician and health care team before you take any herbal supplements in any form, even those that are widely popular and commonly used.

Red Raspberry Leaf Tea derived from the leaves of the red raspberry plant. It has been used for centuries to support respiratory, digestive, and uterine health, particularly during pregnancy and childbearing years. It is known to help strengthen and tone the uterine wall and make it more efficient for contractions.

Peppermint Leaf is helpful in relieving nausea, morning sickness, and flatulence.

Ginger Root helps relieve nausea and vomiting.

Evening Primrose for cervical softening close to delivery.

Food and Herbs to Avoid While Pregnant[8]

---

[8] American Pregnancy Association, "Herbs and Pregnancy," **https://americanpregnancy.org/healthy-pregnancy/is-it-safe/herbs-and-pregnancy/**

While you are pregnant, there are certain food types or kinds of cuisine that you should avoid. The Food and Drug Administration has guidelines for certain food types, for example seafood, because of the high mercury content in fish and other seafood. Besides the high mercury content, there is also the danger of harmful bacteria or viruses contained in certain seafood. In addition, undercooked seafood needs to be completely avoided. Undercooked meat, poultry, and eggs need to be avoided as well. Unpasteurized foods, unwashed fruits and vegetables, alcohol, and certain herbal teas need to be avoided as the effects of some of these on the fetus are still inconclusive in some cases.[9]

The list below, while not totally inclusive, contains some food types that should be avoided, followed by some herbs that might not be safe for a growing fetus.

List of Foods to Avoid While Pregnant
1. Raw meat and seafoods
2. Deli meat (may be contaminated with listeria bacteria which may lead to miscarriage)

---

[9] Mayo Clinic Staff, "Pregnancy Nutrition: Foods to Avoid during Pregnancy," November 30, 2023, **https://www.mayoclinic.org/healthy-lifestyle/pregnancy-week-by-week/in-depth/pregnancy-nutrition/art-20043844**

3. Fish with mercury (usually big fish or canned fish; developmental delays and brain damage associated with mercury)
4. Sushi
5. Raw egg (risk of salmonella)
6. Unpasteurized milk
7. Caffeine
8. Alcohol (fetal alcohol syndrome with developmental delays)
9. Unwashed vegetables (possible contamination with toxoplasmosis)

List of Herbs to Avoid while Pregnant

- Saw palmetto – when used orally, has hormonal activity
- Goldenseal – when used orally, may cross the placenta
- Dong quai – when used orally, due to uterine stimulant and relaxant effects
- Ephedra – when used orally
- Yohimbe – when used orally
- Pau d'arco – when used orally in large doses; contraindicated
- Passionflower – when used orally

- Black cohosh – when used orally in pregnant women who are not at term
- Blue cohosh – when used orally; uterine stimulant can induce labor
- Roman chamomile – when used orally in medicinal amounts
- Pennyroyal – when used orally or topically
- Stay away from cat litter due to the risk of contracting diseases that can be dangerous to the growing fetus

Exercise

Along with a healthy diet, the importance of exercise cannot be overemphasized. There are some light-impact exercises that a knowledgeable trainer or your physician can recommend. A great resource that I found very helpful when I was preparing for both VBACs is Spinning Babies.[10]

Spinning Babies

Spinning Babies is a unique approach to birth created by midwife Gail Tully.

---

[10] Spinning Babies, **https://www.spinningbabies.com/**

This reimagined approach to childbirth describes its process as a physiological approach to preparing for and caring for birth.

The method reasons that during birth, babies descend through the pelvis by turning to fit each curve in the passage. The baby's turns are described as fetal rotations, and the technique argues that if fetal rotations can be made easier, an easier birth can be achieved.

In the next chapter, I will be discussing the different pregnancy trimesters through to the delivery stage. There will be more detailed explanations of what to expect with your doctor's visits.

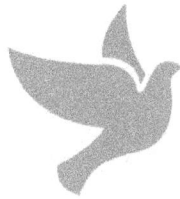

CHAPTER 6

THE PREGNANCY TRIMESTERS

The blessing of the Lord, it maketh rich, and he addeth no sorrow
with it. — Proverbs 10:22 (KJV)

According to the American College of Obstetricians and Gynecologists, a normal pregnancy lasts for about 40 weeks from the first day of your last menstrual period (LMP). Pregnancy is assumed to begin two weeks after the first day of the last menstrual period. Therefore, an extra two weeks is counted at the beginning of your pregnancy when you are actually not pregnant.

Thus, pregnancy officially lasts for ten months, which is 40 weeks, and not nine months as is commonly thought. Typically, your pregnancy is divided into three trimesters that span 40 weeks.

First Trimester: Conception to Week 13

Most women do not find out they are pregnant until the fourth week of gestation. At this juncture, healthy lifestyle habits need to be adopted and it is crucial for smokers and drinkers to quit at this point to avoid harming their baby. All expectant mothers need to start a healthy diet and stop all medications that might be harmful to the baby and consult with a physician to be cleared. Healthy habits are crucial for the development of the fetus since all the organs form in the first trimester. It is also essential to begin taking prenatal vitamins, because vitamins are essential for proper fetal development. For example, folic acid is necessary for neural tube development and a lack or absence can lead to spina bifida.

During the first trimester, you can begin your search for a provider by gathering information and speaking to trusted sources.

Ideally, the time to start looking for providers is when you have a positive pregnancy test and confirmation. However, most providers will not take patients until the 6th week of gestation.

Schedule your initial visit with the obstetrician you select when they will start seeing you, since the first trimester is when your medical history is discussed. This includes questions about family, birth histories, surgical histories, and pregnancy history. This is the time to address all questions and concerns you might have. During the initial visit to your obstetrician, you can also evaluate the rapport you have and decide if this provider is someone you would feel comfortable assisting you with bringing a new life into the world.

The first visit should include blood work (to check for infections like HIV and other STIs as well as your hemoglobin and hepatitis risk or exposure), Pap smear, ultrasound, and assessment of risk for other complications including a miscarriage. Despite a good number of pregnancies ending in a miscarriage — at least an estimated 10 to 20%, according to the Mayo Clinic[11] — miscarriages are not talked about often.

---

[11] Mayo Clinic, "Miscarriage: Overview," September 8, 2023, https://www.mayoclinic.org/diseases-conditions/pregnancy-loss-miscarriage/symptoms-causes/syc-20354298

In most cases, miscarriages occur when the fetus is not compatible, and the body gets rid of it.

A good number of women have had a miscarriage or multiple miscarriages but are reluctant to share their experience because they do not want to seem incapable—even though it is a phenomenon that many women experience.

Shedding the taboo around miscarriages will enable women who have experienced them understand that they are not alone and that they can still conceive and have healthy babies in spite of their medical history.

Oftentimes, bleeding while pregnant is associated with a miscarriage, but there are other common causes of vaginal bleeding caused by other factors:

a. Implantation bleed, where the fertilized egg attaches itself to the lining of the uterus and there is a small bleed that happens 10 to 14 days after conception. Nothing to worry about, but still see your provider to ensure that all is well.

b. Ectopic pregnancy, which is a real and life-threatening emergency. The fertilized egg is implanted outside the uterus, in the ovaries, fallopian tube, or abdomen and can cause life-threatening bleeding. Reach out to your medical care provider if there is any bleeding.

c. Spontaneous miscarriage, in which for some reason, the pregnancy is lost in the first trimester or sometimes in the second.

Most doctors may not do much about vaginal bleeding until week 21 since that is when the pregnancy is considered viable.

Other things to expect include one prenatal visit a month from weeks 4 through 28.

Another important factor to look out for are symptoms of morning sickness. The most common symptoms are nausea and vomiting, which can be relieved using anti-emetic medications.

Some women experience mood swings and food cravings. Reach out to your provider for the best advice if you have these symptoms, as your provider may have to try several medications to find which works best. Getting your posture right is important for the entirety of your pregnancy. Modern culture can encourage being sedentary and this affects pregnancy.

You might be encouraged to use a balance disc wobble cushion as a seat because it helps with core balance and proper posture. This is good for the baby and is recommended by Spinning Babies.

Second Trimester: Week 14 to Week 26

In the second trimester, you will still be meeting with doctors at least once a month. During these visits, you usually will be monitored for weight changes in addition to submitting urine samples to check for infections and glucose in the urine. Protein checks are also done to detect preeclampsia and other risk factors. Weight is an indicator of development of the fetus. Blood pressure checks are also done. Most of the time, a pregnant woman will have a blood pressure lower than that of a non-pregnant woman. The fundal height (the size of the uterus) is checked, and ultrasounds are done to check the anatomy and organs of the growing fetus to ensure that developmental milestones are being reached.

For most women, the second trimester is an enjoyable period because they have usually overcome the hump of morning sickness and started to develop a healthy appetite. They are more settled into the pregnancy.

While this time is a honeymoon period of sorts, women are still encouraged to avoid eating raw foods, drinking alcohol, or using tobacco. The second trimester also brings a lot of bodily changes. These range from breast tenderness, widening hips, and discomfort in the pelvic region due to stretching in the ligament as the fetus gets bigger, to frequent urination due to strain on the bladder, digestive issues such as constipation and acid reflux, and increased weight gain and indigestion. Beginning in the 18th week, the baby's kicks can be felt. For first-time mothers the sensation of kicks may not be immediately apparent since it might be a bit hard to tell what a "normal" kick feels like.

The second trimester is the time to actively start taking steps to ensure a natural delivery. To that end, I would recommend the following considerations.

1. Start doing the activities in Spinning Babies. There are four major maneuvers that Spinning Babies recommends that I found quite helpful. The reason to start these exercises early is so the ligaments can be stretched in readiness for delivery. The first maneuver is the forward leaning inversion, which naturally creates more space for the baby and is recommended

once or twice a week. The second is the side lying release, which helps with pelvic mobility. This maneuver is a team effort and will require assistance from your partner. The third maneuver is the psoas release, which relieves and eliminates lower back and leg pain and helps to release tension in the psoas muscles. The fourth is the abdominal release to help the broad ligament relax, giving the baby more room to get into position for labor.

2. Look into the Bradley Method of childbirth. The Bradley Method focuses on relaxation techniques and teaches you how to manage labor through deep breathing and relaxation. The method is important because learning how to breathe this way is important and will be necessary during labor.

3. Start watching videos and seeking out platforms that offer childbirth classes, prenatal classes. Also seek out positive reinforcement stories from women who have had successful natural deliveries and VBACs.

4. Start working on a birth plan.

5. Reach out to your doula and provider and use them as resources to answer your questions as well as get some tips on how to prepare.

6. Do "Chinese squats" (also known as "Asian squats") and continue doing those Kegel exercises.

Third Trimester: Week 27 – Week 40

Even though the duration for most pregnancies is 40 weeks, the baby is already full term at 37 weeks and can come at any time. A baby born before 37 weeks is called preterm or premature. Doctor visits are still monthly until the 36-week mark.

At week 36, the visits then become weekly and the pelvic checks to measure dilation and the position of the baby will begin. The doctor will also continue to check your blood pressure and weight to ensure both you and the baby are doing well. Urine checks are also done to rule out diabetes and a third trimester ultrasound many be done to rule out any deformities and to make sure the baby is growing normally.

If there are any complications in the pregnancy such as gestational diabetes and signs of preeclampsia or placenta previa, you will have to see the doctor more often since such pregnancies are classified as high risk.

The third trimester is when everything starts to come together and is when the team is solidified. Starting at the 34th or 36th week, your doula can start making visits with you to your doctor, so that the necessary questions can be asked and to serve as an additional set of ears. This is also the time to have your birth plan reviewed with your doctor and making sure every member of your team has a copy and understands what their roles are.

Between Week 36-37, your doctor will check for Group B strep, which is done by swabbing both the vaginal and rectal areas. If positive, antibiotics will be administered before delivery. The purpose for administering antibiotics is to serve as a prophylaxis, since being Group B positive in some instances can expose the baby to the risk of contracting meningitis while passing through the birth canal.

Ultrasounds during the third trimester also confirm the position of the baby in the uterus. It is important to determine if the baby is breech, as this is not favorable for a vaginal delivery; the vertex position is optimal for natural deliveries or VBACs.

If the baby is in a breech position after an ultrasound, this should not be a cause for alarm. The reason for the positioning could be that the position seems comfortable. If the pelvic inlet is not open enough or there is a strained ligament or the pelvic muscles are not relaxed and there is tension, the baby will choose the position that offers optimal comfort. Repositioning can be achieved by performing some exercises from the Spinning Babies technique.

One of the positions suggested by Spinning Babies is the forward leaning inversion, which creates room in the lower uterus and allows the baby to then gravitate naturally towards the lower uterus. Gravity also aids in pulling the baby's head downwards.

At week 36, doing ball stretches and exercises can help you to develop strength.

By week 37, drinking fresh pineapple juice helps to soften the cervix. Women who are diabetic or have been diagnosed with gestational diabetes might need to speak with their physicians first due to the sugar content found in pineapples.

In the third trimester, around week 37, the doctor also starts to check for the softening of the cervix, which is called effacement. The cervix is supposed to thin out as the pregnancy progresses and 100% effacement is typically optimal.

At week 37, the check of dilation, which is the opening of the cervix, is done in conjunction with the effacement check. Dilation and effacement begin once the baby is engaged (engagement refers to the movement of the baby's head down into the pelvis).

Once the baby's head is engaged, dilation and effacement start to progress, and this kick-starts labor. Physically, engagement can be observed by a change in the position of the belly, since it appears to drop because the head of the baby is now downwards.

Another crucial test that is performed is that for the Rh factor. These checks are usually performed in the first and third trimesters.

In the first trimester, if you are Rh negative, RhoGAM is administered via injection to prevent your body from producing antibodies against the next pregnancy. This is also why any bleeding during the pregnancy usually triggers Rh testing, especially if the mother is Rh negative. If you're Rh negative, you will be given RhoGAM medication.

Braxton-Hicks contractions also begin to be felt in the third trimester. These usually are not painful but just involve tightening and relaxing of the uterine wall. Also known as prodromal or false labor pain, it is the body's way of preparing for true labor but does not indicate that labor has actually begun.

The third trimester is also a good time to begin using an app to track the movement of the baby. It is also best to have an app for contractions. Further, it is advisable to talk with your doctor about any pains, aches, or unusual swelling that you experience.

This is also the best time to discuss the use of an epidural with your partner, doula, and doctor. You should gather as much information as possible to make an educated decision about the choice to have an epidural administered. If you decide to not have any epidural administered, that decision should be accompanied by learning breathing techniques that help you with muscle relaxation to manage the pain of labor.

The third trimester is also a good time to begin to put together a hospital bag (see Chapter 8 for a list of what you'll want to include).

The third trimester is a good time to compile a music playlist. Soothing music is helpful in creating a calm environment to facilitate the process of labor. Compile some favorite scripture and motivational quotes to meditate on during the labor process. You might jump-start labor by drinking raspberry leaf tea; this can start as early as week 32.

The recommendation is usually one tea bag twice a day and you can check with retailers on where to purchase these. In addition to the raspberry leaf tea, evening primrose helps to soften the cervix as well. Also, start taking short walks for at least 20 minutes twice a day.

During the third trimester, it is not uncommon for some doctors to back out of a VBAC plan, especially if they feel unprepared or have their confidence tested. Thus, by week 38, some doctors might sound the warning that a cesarean section may be performed if the mother's cervix is not dilating as expected.

Do not let anxiety get the best of you. Stay calm and stick to the plan, especially if you know what your end goal is.

Remember, it is your body, and you need to use your voice. Resist the urge to get cornered by the doctors or derailed from your original intent. Do not feel threatened by a physician who is trying to get you to have your baby born a certain way, especially if that is not what you desire. You also want to make educated and faithful decisions and you need to arm yourself with a wealth of knowledge in order to do make these calls. Remember, *"my people are destroyed for lack of knowledge"* (Hosea 4:6 KJV).

From conception through all the trimesters, you have nurtured your growing baby.

You have taken steps to modify your diet to consume foods that are optimal for your baby's development, developed a new fitness regimen, perhaps taken a childbirth class, created a birth plan, packed your hospital bag, rallied your team, practiced your relaxation techniques, and prepared your birth announcement. You have done the heavy lifting of carrying your growing fetus for almost forty weeks and now you are ready to meet your precious baby.

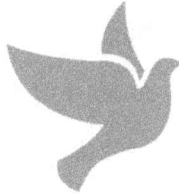

CHAPTER 7

THE DELIVERY

"Shall I bring to the time of birth, and not cause delivery? Says the Lord. "Shall I who cause delivery shut up the womb?" says your God. — Isaiah 66:9 (ESV)

So far, all the steps you have been taking are intended to culminate in a natural birth. This time is very exciting as the mother and family prepare to meet the child. For a first-time mom, the excitement can quickly turn into anxiety as the fear of the unknown looms heavy. For most first-time moms, there is the mistaken assumption that at the fortieth week, labor will just progress naturally, and the baby will be delivered after a few pushes.

However, this time calls for great patience while waiting for labor to naturally progress. By the fortieth week, doctor visits are usually more frequent.

If you have previously had a C-section, there is also a tendency to honestly chicken out at this point and just opt for another cesarean section, because it is somewhat predictable and the feeling of being in control might seem quite appealing.

At this point, doctor visits will mostly center around examining you to assess the positioning of the baby, dilation, effacement, and monitoring to assess if there is engagement of the baby. If the baby is in breech position, some doctors might suggest some form of external manipulation to correct the positioning of the baby or wait an extra week to see if the baby repositions itself naturally. If repositioning does not occur, the next step might be to suggest a cesarean section. This is why Spinning Babies is very important to help with positioning. The most helpful exercise is the forward leaning maneuver, as it has been known to help breech babies change their position. Naturally, after conception, the baby sits upright in the uterus.

Once the delivery time gets closer, the natural process is for the baby to reposition itself and now sit with its head facing downward so that it can engage with the cervix and begin the process of labor.

The failure of the baby to invert itself results in the baby being in breech position. In some cases, the baby may lie in the transverse position, which could also present a barrier to a natural birth and pose a challenge to the mother.

Historically, there were midwives who were skilled in helping to reposition babies, and the process does call for patience on the part of the midwife and a great deal of endurance of the part of the mother, while the baby is massaged into what should be a natural position to begin the labor process. However, with modern conveniences, a more litigious society, a health care system that is frankly in need of repair, and the benefits that accrue to most doctors from scheduling cesarean sections, the surgical option becomes the preferred method of delivery, as it is more controlled and can be scheduled in advance, instead of allowing for the naturally time-consuming process of birth.

Engagement can be measured on a scale of negative five [-5] to plus 3 [+3] stations. Negative five means the baby is not in the pelvic region yet and not engaged, zero [0] means the baby is fully engaged, and plus 3 means the baby is crowning (the top of the baby's head is beginning to emerge from the vaginal opening).

By the 39th to the 40th week, if there is no activity (as measured by the lack of contractions), no sign of labor, or if labor is stalling (measured by a lack of progression in the labor process), the doctor might suggest induction as a next step before a cesarean section is contemplated.

Induction is augmentation of labor. According to the American College of Obstetricians and Gynecologists (ACOG), the goal of induction is to achieve vaginal delivery by stimulating uterine contractions before the spontaneous onset of labor. Essentially, the goal of induction is to kick-start labor. The process is accomplished by administering medications like Cervidil to help soften the cervix and Pitocin to jump-start contractions. With induction, the water might also be broken, which is a stripping of the membrane of the amniotic sac surrounding the baby. Breaking the water is done to help with the progression of labor.

However, according to the ACOG, once the membrane is stripped, there is a window of allowable time within which delivery must occur; otherwise, a cesarean section becomes the next logical step.

Labor is a series of contractions that are progressively more powerful, and that help facilitate cervical dilatation and thinning of the uterus. The process of labor usually starts two weeks before or after the due date. The exact trigger for labor is unknown and every pregnancy is different, just like every woman and her baby are unique. Certain activities such as exercise, sitting on a birthing ball, eating pineapples and such, might help trigger labor. Sex also serves as a trigger for labor since it induces a state of relaxation and the release of the oxytocin hormone, which are optimal for labor to progress.

Every woman experiences labor differently, but there are some common signs that are indicative of labor. For some women, there is a "bloody show," which is a mucus plug tinged with blood. Another sign could be contractions that go from intervals of ten minutes to being progressively more frequent and intense.

It is advisable to have a contraction app to measure contractions or use an old-fashioned timer to measure contractions. Usually if the contractions intensify and are occurring every five minutes or less, it is a sign to alert your birthing team at once. Another sign of being in labor is the rupture of the amniotic sac, typically known as the water breaking. This could be a leak or a big gush of water and is a sign to head down to your chosen birth facility. It is important to take note of the color of the fluid and report this to the doctor or the members of your birthing team.

There are three stages of labor:

1. The first stage is divided into two phases, the latent phase and the active phase. These phases involve dilatation and effacement of the cervix through contractions.

   The latent phase is the longest period and is the time from contraction to being about 4 centimeters dilated. For some women, this stage can take up to a week to complete and is marked by going from 0 centimeters to four centimeters. The active phase of labor is characterized by going from 4 centimeters to 10 centimeters.

2   The second stage of labor is the active pushing and delivery of the baby. This stage can last up to thirty minutes.

3   The third stage of labor is marked by the delivery of the placenta.

My First VBAC Experience

My first VBAC experience was in 2018. My last prenatal visit was at 38 weeks, and thankfully, the baby was vertex and not breech. The Spinning Babies program helped with encouraging mapping, as I tracked my baby's positioning and noticed that he was vertex even as early as the 35th week. I remember talking to the doctor and going over my birth plan. There was no change in my cervix and the doctor noted that if nothing changed in a week, an induction would be scheduled. To prevent a C-section I began walking, stretching on the birthing ball, practicing some Spinning Babies exercises, and drinking pineapple juice. The day before my 39th week appointment, I went to bed as I normally did and was awakened by a sharp and unusual pain. We were two hours away from the doctor I intended to use when I realized thar I was indeed having contractions.

I pulled out my contraction app and began timing the intervals between each contraction and the intensity. The pain was bearable and was occurring at intervals of five minutes.

But since it was so late and we were so far away from the hospital I intended to use, I decided to wait it out. I woke my husband up, but he was so sleepy and suggested we wait until the morning. We waited until about 6 AM., and I got out of bed to get my two older children ready for school, as it was the first day of school.

At this point, the pain became so unbearable that I could hardly stand it. I went to use the toilet and observed a bloody show. At the point I noticed blood, we realized the show was about to begin and we began the long two-hour trek. On the way to the hospital, I called my doula and notified her that the baby was on his way. I called my doctor as well and he advised us to head down to the hospital instead of waiting for my scheduled appointment time that day. Once we got to the hospital I was taken to the labor and delivery triage area. When a cervical check was done, I was only dilated fingertip wide, and the suggestion was to monitor my progression. In an hour I went from being fingertip dilated to 2 centimeters dilated and I was admitted.

My doctor came in about 10:00 a.m. and even though I hadn't dilated beyond 2 centimeters, I was still in active labor.

The doctor tried to break my water and was a bit flustered as he was not able to. He said would allow the labor to progress until I asked for a cesarean section. I felt pressured to give in but realized I had been planning for this moment for months and could not give in now. At this point I felt God's peace come over me. I was also tired and so I decided to take a nap. I had a mobile monitor on, so I did not have to stay in bed. When I decided to lie down, I used the peanut pillow, meditating on God's promises. I then decided to go the restroom and at this point my water broke and I was now 6 centimeters dilated. The pain had progressed in intensity and was quite bad as I had opted for a non-medicated birth. Since this was my first natural delivery, the pain was rather intense, and the duration of labor was also quite long. When I got to 8 centimeters dilated, I requested some medication to take the edge off the pain.

There were several options at this point, a low-dose morphine or nitrogen oxide (commonly referred to as laughing gas), which did absolutely nothing to help with the pain.

The medicine made me drowsy, and I began to have the urge for a bowel movement, but the nurse advised me against that. An urge for a bowel movement was a sign of the baby crowning, as the head of the baby was pushing on the rectum. Additionally, I got a medical episiotomy to lessen the degree of any vaginal wall tearing. Within minutes, I was able to start pushing and in five minutes the baby was delivered. I had my first vaginal birth after two cesarean sections to the glory of God!

My Second VBAC Experience

My second VBAC experience was in 2021. There was a three-year gap between the first and the second and this was not a planned pregnancy. I kept the same routine as with the first VBAC and to be quite honest, I was more relaxed this time as it was not my first rodeo. At the 38th week, just as with my first VBAC, I had not commenced labor. I had the same doula and doctor, and they were quite familiar with me and my needs.

Interestingly, I conceived during the Covid-19 pandemic, and during this time, doulas were restricted from the labor rooms.

At 39 weeks I went to see my doctor and he advised that if I did not go into active labor in four days, he would induce me. I did not want to be induced, but my doctor went ahead and scheduled me for an induction.

It is quite important for pregnant mothers to have open conversations with their doctors even when the doctors make decisions that the mothers are opposed to. I did trust my doctor and his judgment, but still had the urgency to challenge his decision as it was contrary to my desires regarding my choice. It is of utmost importance to note that I am not advocating for or suggesting that you go against medical advice. Rather, I am suggesting that you advocate for yourself and let your voice be heard while still deferring to medical advice and what your physician and medical team believe is best in your unique situation. My doctor and I were able to communicate openly, and I was able to dialogue with him about why I did not want to be induced. Obviously, if he had at any point expressed concern for my life or that of my baby, I would have gladly deferred to his medical advice.

Inductions typically are optimal when the body of the mother is ready. Typically, most inductions proceed with administering oxytocin, and I was concerned about the effects it might have, one of which is possible uterine rupture in patients who have had previous cesarean sections. My doctor suggested that if oxytocin were given, he would give me a low dose, which he was sure my body would be able to handle well.

I went home and prayed about it as was my custom. A day before I was scheduled to be induced, I began contracting. When the intensity increased and the contractions were occurring at five-minute intervals, we made the journey to my doctor to begin the birthing process. This time around, rather than check into the hospital, I checked into a hotel and allowed my labor to progress, staying in touch with my doula the entire time. We agreed that I would go in for my induction on the scheduled day. I went in as scheduled and made my request to not have oxytocin administered. So, alternatively, my doctor broke my water to see if doing so would make the labor progress.

At this point, the contractions became quite intense and the pain intensified. After I labored for about three to four hours, it was time to push, and the baby was delivered.

During the labor process, the pain became quite unbearable, and I requested an epidural, but my doctor was opposed to it as he felt I was close to having the baby and an epidural would have only served to delay the process.

And that was how I had my second vaginal birth after having had two cesarean sections! After months of planning, I now had two babies delivered vaginally after previous cesarean sections. As I cared for my infants, I also had to prioritize nurturing myself. I needed to heal so I could be in the best position to care for my babies and the rest of my family. Looking back on my deliveries, a key component that made the process manageable was having comfort items packed in my hospital bag to create a relaxing environment. I remember playing the game "What's in Your Bag" at baby showers and while some items were absolutely necessary to have, there were some that I could have done without. The next chapter addresses some items I packed. Ultimately, bring along what you believe you do need as you want to make sure your experience is as pleasant as possible.

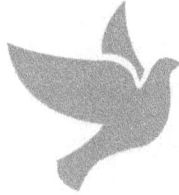

CHAPTER 8

WHAT TO BRING TO THE HOSPITAL

He makes all things beautiful in its time.

— Ecclesiastes 3:11 (NIV)

Preparing to have a baby is very much like planning to go on a journey. With a trip, you choose a destination, map out places of interest, schedule tours, and importantly, pack appropriately. Having a baby also requires that you bring a bag filled with some necessary items. As any seasoned traveler knows, the key is to pack light and avoid bringing unnecessary items. I have attempted to make a list of what I consider essentials that you will most likely need while in the hospital to deliver your baby.

Hospital Bag Checklist for Mom and Dad

- Toothbrush
- Toothpaste
- Body wash, shampoo
- Shaving gel and razor
- Deodorant
- Hair comb/hairbrush
- Hair ties
- Scarves and bonnets
- Underwear and boxers
- Pajamas
- Going-home outfit
- Slippers or comfortable non-slip socks
- Lip balm
- Eyeglasses or contact solution and case
- Phone charger with extra-long (10-foot) cord
- Portable Bluetooth speakers
- Phone, iPad, Kindle, or other electronic devices
- Headphones
- Camera
- Photo props
- Snacks

Mommy's Must-Haves

- Birth plan: Have this handy at all times; review it with your provider, give a copy to the labor and delivery nurses on arrival, and makes sure your team has a copy as well.
- Driver's license and insurance card: To show during registration and the check-in process.
- Comfortable robe: Most hospital gowns are uncomfortable, especially when you're taking laps around the unit.
- Going-home outfit
- Nursing bra and nipple cream
- Comfy slippers
- Have your favorite playlists or podcast readily available
- Portable Bluetooth speakers
- Phone, iPad, Kindle, or other electronic devices
- Headphones
- Phone charger with extra-long cord
- Essential oil and diffuser for a soothing and calming environment.
- Adult diaper or extra-large sanitary pads
- Nursing pillow

- Pillow and blanket
- Snacks: Pack some light snacks you enjoy eating for yourself and your partner. It is likely you will be hungry and worn out post-delivery. Seriously, on multiple occasions after delivery, I was exhausted and hungry and the hospital cafeteria was closed.
- Water and electrolyte-based drink: If you're not able to drink water during labor, having fluids on deck afterwards will be a lifesaver.

Baby Bag Must-Haves

- Cute, comfortable, newborn onesies: I would suggest bringing them in both newborn and 0-3-month sizes in case your baby is much bigger than the average newborn.
- Baby blanket: Your hospital will likely provide a blanket, but you may want to use your own.
- Swaddles
- Baby socks, mittens, and booties
- Hats, bows, and hairbands
- Going-home outfit
- Name sign

- Car seat

Family Bag (Partner's Bag) Must-Haves

- Camera and phone: Do not forget these important items to capture the excitement and share the joyous news!
- MULTIPLE device chargers
- Blanket and pillows: Most hospitals will provide these items to keep your partner cozy.
- Toothbrush and toothpaste just in case you are in for a long night.
- Treats and snacks

Things You Can Leave at Home

- Diapers and wipes: Unless you have a preferred brand, the hospital will send you home with a pack of each.
- Breast pump: If you find that you need a pump during your stay, you can always rent one from the hospital.
- Wedding bands and nice jewelry: I suggest you leave most jewelry pieces at home except if you absolutely need them for pictures. A lot is usually going on at the

hospital while you are having a baby and you do not want to risk misplacing a nice piece of jewelry during such an amazing time in your life.

Now, your baby is here! There is so much buzz and activity as you transition from the hospital to your home, and this is where having a baby differs from going on a trip.

It's a journey nestled within several journeys. Once the birthing journey ends, the journey of nesting and raising your baby begins. Oftentimes, this new phase has its own unique set of challenges but be willing to seek help and ask for support. Remember, it truly does take a village and you can manage the postpartum phase and its set of complications with the proper support.

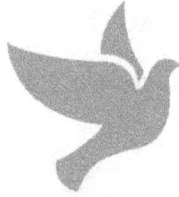

Chapter 9

Postpartum Care and Complications

I have seen something else under the sun: The race is not to the swift or the battle to the strong, nor does food come to the wise or wealth to the brilliant or favor to the learned; but time and chance happen to them all. — Ecclesiastes 9:11 (NIV)]

I just want to congratulate you on your delivery! Great job! Regardless of how you birthed your baby, vaginally or via a cesarean section, childbirth is hard work. Now, it is time for recovery, caring for your body, and nursing yourself back to strength. Following the birth of your baby, you clearly might be vulnerable and in need of help but wanting to show that you can get things done. While it is commendable that you might not want to be a bother to others, you need to take it easy. Childbirth is no easy feat. Your body just carried and gave life to another being. When your body is well rested, you are better able to care for your newborn, so do not burn the candle at both ends.

Ask for and accept all available help. This is not the time to become a supermom; your body needs to heal physically, spiritually, and mentally. Remember, it is perfectly normal to feel overwhelmed and exhausted; it is completely expected. I had body aches for days after my VBACs; it was my body's way of healing from the intense labor. Rest, rest, rest, that's the key! Delegate specific duties to friends and family in order to to give yourself a break. Have helpers on task for duties like cooking, laundry, and watching other children in the house. Put your feet up, you deserve to!

Postpartum Care

After having your baby, you will likely feel sore and need lots of care to feel nurtured as you heal.

Your care should be holistic, and you should attend to your body and mind as you care for sore and perhaps bruised boy parts that need attention.

Breast Care

From the time you deliver, for effective milk production, keep hydrated and drink lots of warm drinks, stay away from cold drinks. To prevent engorgement, massage breasts gently with warm towel compress and express milk frequently, either directly feeding your infant every two hours or using a breast pump.

Use lanolin cream ointment on your breasts to prevent nipple cracking.

Digestive Care

Since pain medication often can lead to constipation, you will need stool softeners and laxatives:

Keeping bisacodyl oral tablets, magnesium hydroxide, 8.6 milligram sennosides, and 100 milligrams docusate sodium tablets will be helpful to make using the bathroom one less hassle to worry about. For bloating and gas, use simethicone 180 milligram tablets as needed.

Perineal and Hemorrhoidal Care

- Hydrocortisone (rectal) 25 milligrams as needed for hemorrhoids
- Witch hazel (Tucks pads) rectally
- Benzocaine-methanol topical spray to use as needed for perineal discomfort
- Cool pack for the perineum area
- It is also perfectly fine to use incontinence pads if needed. I used Depends underwear while postpartum and found them helpful.
- Use sitz baths as needed. These can be purchased before you get to the hospital, as some hospitals may not provide you with one. The benefits include helping with healing if there are vaginal tears and easing perineal discomfort.

Postpartum Complications

Having a baby is a life-changing experience that can be difficult and exhausting. As much as having a baby brings a great deal of excitement, it is also quite a stressful time for most moms and could be fraught with joy, fear, and anxiety, irrespective of the stage in life or age. People experience a range of changes after having a baby, and these emotional, hormonal, financial, physical, and social changes can impact not just new mothers, but fathers, surrogates, and adoptive parents.

Postpartum Depression

Experiencing feelings of having the blues affects up to 75% of women after delivery. At least 15% of these women will develop postpartum depression.[12] For some moms, the feeling of having the blues — which can include mood swings, crying spells, anxiety, and difficulty sleeping — soon quickly passes.

---

[12] Cleveland Clinic, "Postpartum Depression," April 12, 2022, https://my.clevelandclinic.org/health/diseases/9312-postpartum-depression; Mayo Clinic Staff, "Postpartum Depression," November 24, 2022, https://www.mayoclinic.org/diseases-conditions/postpartum-depression/symptoms-causes/syc-20376617

But for others, that feeling lingers and the joy that a new baby should bring is absent as this period is fraught with a severe and unexplained sadness that just does not seem to pass and is medically diagnosed as postpartum depression.

According to the Mayo Clinic, this severe long-lasting form of depression is known as postpartum depression and in most cases, the onset of symptoms occurs within the first two to three days after delivery and may last for up to two weeks.

In some instances, the onset of symptoms occurs even before the birth of the baby and is referred to as peripartum depression. In extremely rare instances, a mood disorder called postpartum psychosis may develop after childbirth.

Symptoms of postpartum depression can occur in even relatively healthy moms and should not be viewed as a character flaw or a sign of some form of weakness. Instead, these symptoms should be addressed as a complication of having given birth. Not to be confused with just simply having baby blues, symptoms of postpartum depression are more intense and could last for months.

In some instances, these symptoms interfere with the ability to take care of the baby and handle other daily needed tasks.

Most mothers struggling with postpartum depression go undiagnosed, either because their symptoms are mistaken for "baby blues," or they do not share their symptoms because of the stigma surrounding mental illness and the fear that disclosure may lead to abandonment and a lack of support. If you experience any symptoms of the blues that persist for more than two weeks, please get help.

Symptoms of Postpartum Depression

Symptoms could last for a few days to a week or even longer after the baby is born and may include:

- Depressed mood or severe mood swings
- Intense irritability and anger
- Crying excessively
- Extreme unexplained sadness
- Loss of appetite
- Reduced concentration
- Withdrawing from support systems such as friends and family

- Severe anxiety and panic attacks

- Hopelessness

- Trouble sleeping

- Restlessness

- Overwhelming tiredness or loss of energy

- Concern about poor mothering skills

- Feelings of worthlessness, shame, guilt, or inadequacy

- Thoughts of harming yourself or your baby

- Feeling overwhelmed

- Recurring thoughts of suicide or death

- Reduced ability to think clearly, concentrate, or make decisions

Factors that Increase Risk of Postpartum Depression

Certain physiological, obstetric, biological, social, and lifestyle factors can put some women at risk for postpartum depression:

- A previous history of depression and anxiety

- Negative attitude towards pregnancy

- Past sexual abuse

- High-risk pregnancies requiring hospitalization

- Young age of the mother during pregnancy

- Hormonal imbalances

- Lack of social support

- Dietary patterns, sleep status, exercise, and physical activities

Diagnosis and Tests

There is no specific test to diagnose postpartum depression, however, your healthcare provider can evaluate you on your postpartum visit to screen for depression. Your provider may do a screening by asking you questions to assess if you have postpartum depression. Be transparent and honest with your provider to enable them to have an accurate picture of your emotions and thoughts.

Management and Treatment

Psychosocial and psychological therapy is the first line of treatment for women with depression. Usually, a combination of therapy and antidepressant drugs is recommended for women, but lactating mothers should be aware of the risks of antidepressant use during breastfeeding and the risk of leaving the disease untreated.

Postpartum Psychosis

Postpartum psychosis is a psychiatric emergency with a potential risk of suicide and infanticide. Postpartum psychosis can affect any new mother. The condition is reversible but quite severe and affects women after they give birth. It is also quite rare but very dangerous. Postpartum psychosis is a mental health emergency and mothers who suffer are at a much higher risk of harming themselves, dying by suicide, or harming their children. If you have symptoms of postpartum psychosis or notice the symptoms in a new mother, please seek help or encourage the woman who seems like she might be at risk to seek help immediately. Although the symptoms of postpartum psychosis might seem similar to those for postpartum depression, they are often more heightened and include:

- Having delusions and hallucinations
- Attempting to self-harm or harm your baby
- Feelings of paranoia
- Excessive outbursts of energy
- Feelings of anger or rage
- Having obsessive thoughts about your baby
- Feeling lost and confused

There are a host of other postpartum complications.

If at any time you begin to experience chest pain, headaches, dizziness, shortness of breath, or any other unusual symptoms, contact your provider immediately and seek emergency help, as these signs could indicate life threatening complications of pregnancy.

Black Mothers and Maternal Mortality

A maternal death is defined by the World Health Organization as "the death of a woman while pregnant or within 42 days of termination of the pregnancy, irrespective of the duration and site of the pregnancy, from any cause related to or aggravated by the pregnancy or its management, but not from accidental or incidental causes."

With a maternal mortality rate that is the highest of any developed nation in the world and more than double the rate of peer countries, the United States is facing a maternal health crisis.[13] Common causes of these deaths include excessive bleeding, infection, heart disease, suicide, and drug overdose.

---

[13] White House Blueprint for Addressing the Maternal Health Crisis, June 2022, https://www.whitehouse.gov/wp-content/uploads/2022/06/Maternal-Health-Blueprint.pdf

Maternal mortality rates are the number of maternal deaths per 100,000 live births. In the United States, rates for Black women were significantly higher than rates for white and Hispanic women.

The rates increased with maternal age and the rate for women aged 40 and over was 6.8 times higher than the rate for women under age 25.[14] Further, southern states in the United States had higher maternal mortality across all races and ethnic groups but especially for Black women.[15]

According to the US Centers for Disease Control, Black women are three times more likely to die from a pregnancy-related cause than white women. Factors contributing to this disparity include variations in the quality of healthcare, underlying chronic conditions, structural racism, and implicit bias.

---

[14] Maternal Mortality Rates 2021, US Centers for Disease Control, https://www.cdc.gov/nchs/data/hestat/maternal-mortality/2021/maternal-mortality-rates-2021.htm#:~:text=In%202021%2C%201%2C205%20women%20died,20.1%20in%202019%20(Table)

[15] White House Blueprint for Addressing the Maternal Health Crisis, https://www.whitehouse.gov/wp-content/uploads/2022/06/Maternal-Health-Blueprint.pdf

A National Bureau of Economic Research study of infants born to first-time mothers from 2007 to 2016 in California showed that for an affluent country, the United States is a risky place for a newborn.

However, the risk is not equally borne by all babies. In the United States, more affluent mothers and their babies are likely to survive the year after childbirth, except when the family is Black. Research has shown that Black mothers and babies have the worst childbirth outcomes in the United States.[16] Research has also found that "maternal mortality rates were just as high among affluent Black women as among low-income white women, so wealth did not shield Black women from maternal mortality. Infants born to the richest Black women tended to have more risk factors, including being born premature or underweight, than those born to the poorest white mothers."[17] The study concluded that the harm to Black mothers and their babies began before birth regardless of socioeconomic class.[18]

---

[16] "Childbirth is Deadlier for Black Families Even When They're Rich, Expansive Study Finds ," *The New York Times,* February 12, 2023, **https://www.nytimes.com/interactive/2023/02/12/upshot/child-maternal-mortality-rich-poor.html**

[17] *Ibid.*

[18] *Ibid.*

While this study was done in California, the Black mothers are still at risk across the United States. In the end, the study concluded that maternal deaths of Black mothers was not about biology or race, but rather about racism.

There was clear evidence to show that irrespective of socioeconomic status, Black patients experienced racism in health care settings and further in childbirth Black mothers are treated differently and given different access to interventions.[19] To unravel the entrenched racism that is so deeply ingrained in the health care system, advocacy for reform and education are essential as well as diversifying the health care workforce and providing Black moms with culturally sensitive care.[20] Reforming the system includes expanding access to midwives and doulas as women who receive care from midwives or doulas were less likely to have preterm birth and cesarean sections and were more likely to breastfeed their babies.[21]

---

[19] *Ibid.*

[20] Annalies Winny and Rachel Bervell, "How Can We Solve the Black Maternal Health Crisis?" *Public Health On Call*, Johns Hopkins Bloomberg School of Public Health, May 12, 2023, **https://publichealth.jhu.edu/2023/solving-the-black-maternal-health-crisis**

[21] *Ibid.*

Doulas are nonclinical, trained health care workers who support pregnant women before, during, and after pregnancy. Compared with clinical providers doulas spend more time supporting their clients and provide extremely beneficial services.

The American College of Obstetricians and Gynecologists credited the continuous presence of a doula during pregnancy as one of the most important tools to improve labor and delivery outcomes.[22] Current research has shown that the accompanying stress that comes with exposure to racism negatively impacts birth outcomes. Thus, it is important to engage the services of doulas during the prenatal period to improve racial disparities by ensuring that Black mothers receive the support they need. Engaging a doula during the prenatal period can be effective in supporting pregnant women in making informed health choices during their pregnancies that in turn result in a lesser likelihood of having a cesarean birth and using pain medication and having shorter labors, more spontaneous births, and greater satisfaction with

[22] "Safe Prevention of the Primary Cesarean Delivery," *American Journal of Obstetrics & Gynecology,* 210(3), March 2014, p. 179-193, https://www.ajog.org/article/S0002-9378(14)00055-6/fulltext

their birthing experience. This is because these women are less likely to have preterm deliveries, low birth weight babies, or suffer from postpartum depression.

A key reason is they are allowed greater agency in the decision-making process, which improves health outcomes.[23]

Infertility

Getting to decide what type of delivery to opt for assumes that there is a pregnancy. For some women the choice may not come for a while or at all as they struggle with infertility. Infertility is defined as not being able to conceive after having consistent unprotected sex for twelve months. Walking through infertility may be some of the hardest journeys some women will have to work through and the pain of trying to conceive can be harrowing as it can be a lonely journey that is filled with feelings of shame and inadequacy over one's body failing to function at doing what should seemingly be such a natural task. The most obvious symptom of infertility is not being able to get pregnant.

[23] Alexis Robles-Fradet and Mara Greenwald, "Doula Care Improves Health Outcomes, Reduces Racial Disparities and Cuts Cost," National Health Law Program, August 8, 2022, **https://healthlaw.org/doula-care-improves-health-outcomes-reduces-racial-disparities-and-cuts-cost/**

However, some women may experience irregular or absent periods. In men, symptoms may be less obvious but hormonal changes that affect sexual function or hair growth can be signs worth investigating further.

For women, certain factors that might affect infertility include:

- Being over age 35
- Having painful periods
- Absent or irregular periods
- A diagnosis of endometriosis or pelvic inflammatory disease
- Have undergone treatment for cancer
- A family or known history of infertility

Infertility occurs more commonly than most probably think and you're not alone in your journey. Several women in the Bible were faced with this challenge and were finally able to conceive, and thankfully, today, there are resources to help women and couples walking the same path.

Whether you are on the journey of trying to conceive or have had your babies and are struggling, I hope you are encouraged to seek help.

Talk with your health care provider, a licensed therapist, or trusted family and friends. You should not suffer alone. Seek help and seek it early.

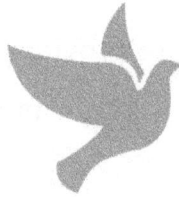

CHAPTER 10

CONCLUSION

Many are the plans in the mind of a man, but it is the purpose of the Lord that will stand. — Proverbs 19:21 [ESV]

The journey from conception to birth will always be one that is clouded with unknowns. Interestingly and quite sadly, humans may never get to fully experience God's highest good and his perfect plan for procreation as one of the curses that resulted from the fall in the Garden of Eden was pain during childbirth. Speaking about God, the scripture reads, to the woman, *"I will surely multiply your pain in childbearing; in pain you shall bring forth children"* (Genesis 3:16 ESV).

In some other versions of the Bible, that same scripture reads, *"I will intensify your labor pains; you will bear children with painful effort"* (CSB), *"I will make your pregnancy very painful"* (CEB), *"You will suffer terribly when you give birth"* (CEV), *"I will multiply thy sorrows, and thy conceptions"* (DRA), *"I will intensify your labor pains; you will bear children in anguish"* (HCSB), *"Multiplying I multiply thy sorrow and thy conception, in sorrow dost thou bear children"* (YLT).

Thus, from quite early on, the beauty of bringing a new life into the world was tainted from the point of conception all the way to birth. Thus, it is no wonder the maternal journey is laced with challenges from infertility all the way to mortality during the birthing process. We are left to wonder what the path to procreation might have looked like without the brokenness of sin, but since we have no clear answers but only the consequences of the Fall, we have to find best practices to manage procreation and ease the process of childbirth in spite of the many pitfalls that loom.

In spite of the pangs that come with childbirth, sometimes requiring surgical intervention, childbearing can still be a positive experience and should not be approached with fear. For most women, being pregnant brings a host of anxieties.

There is concern about diet and which foods to eat or abstain from, concerns about how much physical exertion is appropriate, sleep patterns, and a host of other maladies that come with birthing a new life. Being aware of the challenges that come with pregnancies is useful, as knowing allows room to prepare for the challenges that come. Nonetheless, in spite of how prepared a future mother is, each pregnancy journey is quite unique, and God still ultimately guides and directs the outcome.

Let Jesus be at the center of your journey and trust Him through it all, because all things are possible with him. Remember that you are fearfully and wonderfully made and as long as it is medically safe, you have the right to choose and to not be cornered into doing something you do not want to do. Knowledge is power. And in the end, God's counsel is what stands.

"Unless the Lord builds the house, those who build it labor in vain. Unless the Lord watches over the city, the watchman stays awake in vain. It is in vain that you rise up early and go late to rest, eating the bread of anxious toil; for he gives to his beloved sleep.

Behold, children are a heritage from the Lord, the fruit of the womb a reward. Like arrows in the hand of a warrior are the children of one's youth. Blessed is the man who fills his quiver with them! He shall not be put to shame when he speaks with his enemies in the gate." — Psalm 127 ESV

PRAYER POINTS FOR A VICTORIOUS PREGNANCY AND DELIVERY

1. Thank God and praise God for the gift of the fruit of the womb.

   "Lo, children are a heritage of the LORD: and the fruit of the womb is his reward." — Psalm 127:3 KJV

2. Give thanks and praises to God for conception.

   "Before I formed you in the womb I knew you; Before you were born I sanctified you; I ordained you a prophet to the nations." — Jeremiah 1:5 NKJV

3. Give praises and thanks to God for all three trimesters and for a safe delivery.

4. Pray for God's forgiveness and mercies.

   "Have mercy upon me, O God, according to thy lovingkindness: according unto the multitude of thy tender mercies blot out my transgressions." — Psalm 51:1 KJV

5. Confess in the name of Jesus that all is well with you and the baby inside your womb.

   "I will praise you, for I am fearfully and wonderfully made." — Psalm 139:14 NKJV

6. I profess that the blood of Jesus Christ mixes with my blood to make everything in my body perfect. I soak myself, baby, and family with the blood of Jesus Christ.

7. I receive the strength of the Lord to carry to term and deliver safely.

8. Confess in the name of Jesus that all diseases that accompany pregnancy are not your portion in Jesus Christ's Name.

   "The blessing of the Lord makes one rich, and He adds no sorrow with it." — Proverbs 10:22 NJKV

9. Pray for only the counsel of God to stand concerning the time from conception to delivery.

10. That Jesus Christ will be at the Center of it all, and that you will see His glory and in return, give all the praise to Him. Amen.

Experiencing the birth of a baby can be an extremely joyous event. Thus, wherever you might be on the journey to motherhood, from trying to conceive to perhaps managing the type of delivery experience you might have, the path can often be filled with several unknowns, but God promises to lead us when we fully trust Him. God is interested in procreation and the proliferation of the human species because we are so carefully crafted in His image and after His very likeness. It is my hope that this book helps you pursue God's highest best for you as you are guided by sound medical advice. Importantly, I hope each woman who picks up this book is not only assured of her worth, but comforted in the truth that she has value no matter how her babies are born.

"Behold, children are the heritage from the Lord, the fruit of the womb a reward."

— Psalm 127:3 *ESV*

Glossary

Android pelvis: This type of pelvis bears more resemblance to the male pelvis. It is narrower than the gynecoid pelvis and is shaped more like a heart or a wedge.

Anthropoid pelvis: An anthropoid pelvis is narrow and deep. Its shape is similar to an upright egg or oval.

Antiemetic: Medicine used to treat nausea and vomiting.

Bradley Method: According to the American Academy of Husband-Coached Childbirth (AAHCC), the purpose of the Bradley Method is to teach "natural birth and view birth as a natural process." In this method, the conditions essential for a laboring woman are darkness, solitude, quiet, physical comfort during the first stage of labor, physical relaxation, controlled breathing, and the need for closed eyes or appearance of sleep.

Braxton-Hicks contractions: Braxton-Hicks contractions, also known as prodromal or false labor pains, are contractions of the uterus that typically are not felt until the second or third trimester of the pregnancy. Braxton-Hicks contractions are the body's way of preparing for true labor, but they do not indicate that labor has begun.

Breech position: The breech position is when a baby is positioned feet or bottom first in the uterus. Ideally, a baby is positioned so that the head is delivered first during a vaginal birth.

Cervidil: A medication delivered through a vaginal insert. It assists with labor by softening the cervix and preparing it for birth. Cervidil is the only FDA-approved vaginal insert for cervical ripening.

Cesarean section, C-section, or Cesarean birth: The surgical delivery of a baby through a cut (incision) made in the mother's abdomen and uterus. Health care providers use it when they believe it is safer for the mother, the baby, or both.

Doula: A woman, typically without formal obstetric training, who is employed to provide guidance and support to a pregnant woman during labor.

Dural sac: The membranous sac that encases the spinal cord within the bony structure of the vertebral column.

Epidural: An injection given in the patient's back to stop the feeling of pain in parts of the body.

Epidural space: A tissue plane between the dura mater, covering the spinal nerve and dural sac, and the periosteum and ligaments within the vertebral canal and the intervertebral foramen.

Fundal height: The distance from the pubic bone to the top of the uterus measured in centimeters. After 24 weeks of pregnancy, fundal height often matches the number of weeks you have been pregnant.

Gestational diabetes: A type of diabetes that can develop during pregnancy in women who do not already have diabetes.

Gynecoid pelvis: The most common type of pelvis in females, generally considered to be the typical female pelvis. Its overall shape is round, shallow, and open.

Lumbar puncture: A procedure where a health care provider inserts a hollow needle into the space surrounding the spinal column in the lower back to withdraw some cerebrospinal fluid or insert medicine.

Morning sickness: Extreme, excessive nausea and vomiting during pregnancy.

Mucus plug: A thick piece of mucus that blocks the opening of the cervix during pregnancy.

NICU (neonatal intensive care unit): A hospital ward or department equipped and staffed to provide intensive care to dangerously ill or premature newborn babies.

Pitocin: A synthetic version of oxytocin used as an intravenous medication for labor induction. The drug helps imitate natural labor and birth by causing the uterus to contract.

Platypelloid pelvis. The platypelloid pelvis is also called a flat pelvis. This is the least common type. It is wide but shallow, and it resembles an egg or oval lying on its side.

Prenatal: Before birth; during or relating to pregnancy

Primigravida: A woman who is pregnant for the first time.

Preeclampsia: A serious condition that can develop after the 20th week of pregnancy or after giving birth (called postpartum preeclampsia). In addition to causing high blood pressure, it can cause other major organs like the kidneys and liver to malfunction.

Rh: The Rh factor is a protein that can be found on the surface of red blood cells. If your blood cells have this protein, you are Rh positive and if your blood cells do not have this protein, you are Rh negative.

RhoGAM: A prescription medicine given by intramuscular injection that is used to prevent Rh immunization, a condition in which an individual with Rh-negative blood develops antibodies after exposure to Rh-positive blood.

Spinal anesthesia: A neuraxial anesthesia technique in which local anesthetic is placed directly in the intrathecal space (subarachnoid space). The subarachnoid space houses sterile cerebrospinal fluid, the clear fluid that bathes the brain and spinal cord.

Transverse position: When a baby is positioned sideways, lying horizontal across the uterus, rather than vertical.

Trial of labor after Cesarean Section (TOLAC): Referred to as an attempt at vaginal delivery in women with previous cesarean sections. Successful TOLAC is defined as spontaneous or instrumental (assisted by vacuum or forceps) delivery in a woman undergoing TOLAC. Unsuccessful TOLAC is defined as failure to achieve VBAC in women undergoing TOLAC resulting in emergency cesarean section.

Unpasteurized: Foods in raw form that have not been exposed to high temperatures or treated to kill harmful microbes and are associated with increased risk of foodborne infections.

VBAC: Vaginal birth after cesarean delivery

Vertex: Means "crown of the head." This means that the crown of the fetus's head is presenting towards the cervix.

Abbreviations for Versions of the Bible

CEV – Contemporary English Version

CSB – Christian Standard Bible

DBA – Douay-Rheims Bible

ESV – English Standard Version

HCSB – Holman Christian Standard Bible

KJV – King James Version

NKJV – New King James Version

NIV – New International Version

YLT – Young's Literal Translation

www.ingramcontent.com/pod-product-compliance
Lightning Source LLC
Chambersburg PA
CBHW030006110426
42736CB00040BA/528